The Source for Syndromes

Gail J. Richard

Debra Reichert Hoge

> Skills: Speech and Language
> Ages: Birth through 18

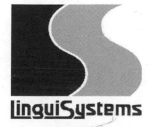

LinguiSystems

LinguiSystems, Inc.
3100 4th Avenue
East Moline, IL 61244-9700

1-800 PRO-IDEA
1-800-776-4332

FAX: 1-800-577-4555
E-mail: service@linguisystems.com
Web: www.linguisystems.com

TDD: 1-800-933-8331
         (for those with hearing impairments)

About the Authors

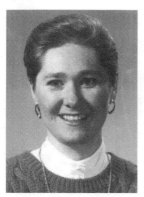

Gail J. Richard

Gail J. Richard, Ph.D., CCC/SLP, is a professor in the Department of Communication Disorders and Sciences at Eastern Illinois University in Charleston. Her responsibilities include undergraduate and graduate courses and clinical supervision in the clinic. Her areas of expertise focus on childhood and adolescent language disorders, such as autism, selective mutism, language processing, learning disabilities, and other developmental disorders. Gail's experience prior to joining the university faculty included public school therapy and a diagnostic/therapeutic preschool setting. Gail consults with school districts on a regular basis to problem-solve and assist in educational programming ideas for special needs students. She is a popular presenter for workshops around the country due to the practical nature of the information she shares with her audiences.

Gail's professional honors and awards include Past President and Fellow of the Illinois Speech-Language-Hearing Association, recipient of the Illinois Clinical Achievement Award, Outstanding Alumnus Award at Southern Illinois University-Carbondale, member of the American Speech-Language-Hearing Association's (ASHA's) Legislative Council, five Faculty Excellence Awards, and NCAA Faculty Athletics Representative for Eastern Illinois University. Previous publications with LinguiSystems include *The Source for Autism* and *The Language Processing Test* and *Language Processing Kit*, co-authored with Mary Anne Hanner.

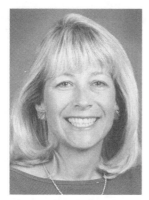

Debra Reichert Hoge

Debra Reichert Hoge, Ed.D., CCC/SLP, is an associate professor in the Department of Special Education and Communication Disorders at Southern Illinois University in Edwardsville. She teaches undergraduate and graduate courses in early intervention, child language development and disorders, and low incidence populations. She also teaches early childhood special education courses. Prior to becoming a faculty member at Southern Illinois, Debra taught in the public schools and at a center for autism. Debra has presented numerous workshops throughout the country on early intervention; assessment and intervention with infants, toddlers, and their families; and early childhood special education issues. She was chosen as an author and presenter on two national inservice grants awarded to the American Speech-Language-Hearing Association (ASHA): ASHA's Building Blocks and ASHA's Interdisciplinary Preschool Project.

Debra is a native and lifelong resident of St. Louis, Missouri, and lives there with her husband, James, and daughter, Jillian Jean. *The Source for Syndromes* is Debra's first publication with LinguiSystems.

Dedication

To our families, for their support and encouragement during the completion of this project; and to the children and their families with whom we interact each day, for challenging and inspiring us!

Table of Contents

Introduction

" The doors of wisdom are never shut. "
Benjamin Franklin

Are you feeling challenged to stay current in your clinical practice?

Do you feel like one more new, fancy term introduced at a staffing will be the final straw?

Are you stressed by the complexity of children appearing in early intervention settings?

Are you tired of reading theory?

Do you wish someone would tell you what to do with a specific child tomorrow?

> The nature of disorders evidenced in preschool children today is very different than it was five or ten years ago.

Sorry, there is no magic solution. It would be nice if someone could prescribe two aspirin and bed rest for what ails you. Unfortunately the dilemmas facing practitioners today are a bit more involved than a simple aspirin can cure, but aspirin might help your headache!

The nature of disorders evidenced in preschool children today is very different than five or ten years ago. Students enrolled in early intervention programs today do not display simple language delays from poor stimulation or otitis media. Preschool teachers and adjunct professionals are astounded by the never-ending challenges entering their doors for services. Are incidence figures increasing, or is it our imagination? They are definitely increasing. Why? There are a few theories being proposed that probably each contribute in part.

- **Improved education and awareness of disabilities**
  Parents and professionals are constantly exposed to new information from a variety of media options. Resources are readily available to consumers and professionals at the click of a mouse. Information access has been streamlined by modern technology. Investigative news programs and magazines love a human interest story that involves a family's struggles to help their child. Introduction to disabilities and treatments comes to the public at a steady pace each day.

- **Changes in diagnostic criteria**
  The *Diagnostic and Statistical Manual of Mental Disorders, Fourth Edition* (1994) modified criteria in many of the Clinical Disorders on Axis I to better coincide with clinical presentation of these disorders. Consistency across settings was insured by correlating with the International Classification of Diseases (ICD). Delineation of characteristics in *DSM-IV* allowed professionals in an educational setting to apply the criterion more reliably for referral to specialists for diagnosis. The language of diagnosis became more "user friendly" and less incomprehensible and austere.

- **Stresses to neurological integrity of DNA**
  Some research studies have suggested slight changes in the neurological code passed to the next generation as a result of exposure to environmental factors, such as chemicals, power lines, toxic wastes, radiation, etc. In addition, a few genetic studies show traits becoming more pronounced in each successive generation. For example, an obsessive-compulsive disorder in a father becomes Asperger's syndrome in his daughter; a speech-language delay in the daughter is later evidenced as a language-learning disability in her child. These links are difficult to substantiate and they require careful study over time, but anecdotal data continues to strengthen while the studies are being conducted.

- **Increase in infant survival rates for medically-fragile cases**
  Improvements in medical technology have decreased infant fatalities due to complicating medical conditions. Many babies whose neurological deficits would have been terminal in the past now survive. Parents and professionals are faced with numerous issues in attempting to foster the development of these children.

Despite better education, awareness, and medical technology, meeting the diverse and expanding needs of young children today is a complex challenge! The acquisition rate of medical knowledge continues to increase with combined efforts. Definitive answers to DNA coding and causes of disabilities will probably be discovered within our lifetime, yet the answers to clinical questions of how to deliver appropriate services on a daily basis never seem to be provided.

That's the reason for *The Source for Syndromes*. Expending energy and time tracking down definitions for a fancy label on a preschool child often results in extreme frustration. Citations from medical literature rarely address what the primary speech-language characteristics are and where to start intervention efforts. This book attempts to summarize pertinent information in one place for the practicing professional. It also encourages the professional to move beyond the label to see a child with specific symptoms that can be addressed in early intervention.

The Source for Syndromes is designed for the practicing speech-language pathologist. The syndrome disabilities included are approached from a perspective of intervention. The book is NOT intended to be a definitive, extensive current review of medical research on cause. Our purpose is to delineate the nature of each syndrome as clearly as possible and to indicate the primary remediation focus for speech-language pathologists.

Each syndrome chapter is divided into five sections:

- Syndrome Definition

- Behavioral Characteristics Profile

- Speech-Language Issues

- Intervention Issues

- Summary Comments

The Source for Syndromes will help the practicing professional gain a global understanding of the primary disability identified, focus on the pertinent speech-language characteristics, and generate goals and strategies to begin intervention efforts at a preschool level.

So don't become overwhelmed by the challenges presented. You might be surprised by how much you already know and reaffirmed by what you read. Benjamin Franklin knew that the learning process never stops and encouraged us to keep the doors wide open. We hope *The Source for Syndromes* will make the journey less arduous and somewhat enjoyable!

This book helps you:

- gain a global understanding of specific syndromes

- focus on pertinent speech-language characteristics

- generate goals and strategies to begin intervention efforts at a preschool level

Angelman Syndrome

Characteristics

- Developmental delays/Severe cognitive impairment
- Epilepsy/Seizure disorder
- Distinctive facial and physical characteristics
- Unusual physical movements
- Feeding and swallowing difficulties
- Short attention span
- Behaviors related to educational planning

- non-progressive, genetic, neurological disorder

- 1/10,000 to 1/25,000 live births

- limited expressive language

- oral-motor dysfunction

- the "happy puppet" syndrome

Syndrome Definition

Angelman syndrome is a non-progressive neurological disorder first reported by Dr. Harry Angelman in 1965 in England (Miles, 1997). Originally, Angelman syndrome was thought to be rare, but current incidence figures range from one in 10,000 live births to one in 25,000 (Miles, 1997). This syndrome is also known as the "happy puppet" syndrome due to the puppet-like arm postures and typically smiling facial expressions (Shprintzen, 1997).

The cause of Angelman syndrome in at least 50% of the cases is a deletion from chromosome 15; a small piece of the chromosome is actually missing (Shprintzen, 1997). Although parents are not considered "carriers" of Angelman syndrome, the deletion usually arises from the mother's chromosome. If the deletion on chromosome 15 is from the father, Prader-Willi syndrome will result (see Prader-Willi Syndrome, pp. 90-97). In most of the families, only one individual is affected by Angelman syndrome. Current thoughts on the importance of the genes on chromosome 15 include the possibility that the development of parts of the brain, particularly those parts associated with language and movement, is carried on these genes. The partial deletion affecting the chromosome results, therefore, in lack of development of these brain areas.

Angelman syndrome may be unrecognized at birth and may not be diagnosed until the early childhood years when associated behaviors become apparent. The diagnosis is usually made by a pediatrician or a geneticist. There is currently no prenatal diagnostic test available, and routine genetic testing may not detect Angelman syndrome. A blood test called a *fluorescent in situ hybridization (FISH)* test is currently the most accurate genetic test. This is a test of the DNA to detect the gene deletion.

Behavioral Characteristics Profile . . . .

The primary characteristics and behaviors are summarized in the chart on page 9 and explained in the following information. The behavioral characteristics associated with Angelman syndrome may not be seen in every child affected by the syndrome.

Developmental Delays

Children with Angelman syndrome are often initially diagnosed due to their delay in general development. Of particular note are delays in meeting motor milestones (i.e., sitting and walking) and in speech development. The pediatrician and family may be the first persons to note the delays in development. As these children develop, severe learning disabilities become apparent, with most of these children testing in the severe range of mental retardation. It is thought that the hyperactivity and short attention span may play a factor in the impaired learning abilities exhibited by members of this population.

Epilepsy/Seizure Disorder

Approximately 80% of children with Angelman syndrome also exhibit seizures, according to Miles (1997). Abnormal EEGs have also been noted in these children, and anticonvulsant medications are widely used to control the seizure behaviors.

Facial Features

Children with Angelman syndrome show a large, wide, smiling mouth with widely-spaced or irregular teeth. *Macrostomia* is a term used for "wide mouth." The upper lip may be thin, and there may be a tendency to hold the tongue between the lips. An open mouth at rest has also been noted, as well as the presence of tongue thrust. Deep-set eyes have been noted, and a prominent chin may also be seen. This prominent chin may be referred to as *mandibular protrusion* and may be related to the oral-motor movements noted in Angelman syndrome.

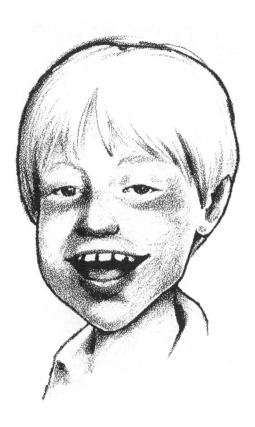

Physical Features

Microcephaly (below-average head size) with flattening in the back or occiput area has been noted in Angelman syndrome. Another physical feature is the characteristic gait used by these children, which is wide-based and stiff-legged.

Hypopigmentation of the skin, which results in very fair complexions, fair hair, and blue eyes, is characteristic in 60% of children with Angelman syndrome. These children sunburn easily; parents or caregivers must protect these children's skin when they are outdoors.

Visual disturbances in the mild range have been estimated in 40% of this population. Squinting, nystagmus (roving eye movements), optic atrophy, strabismus, and poor eyesight have been found in children with Angelman syndrome. Scoliosis has also been found in a small number of these children.

Movement Patterns

Unusual movement patterns have been noted in Angelman syndrome. Hand flapping, fine tremors, and jerky limb movements have all been observed. These movements are not thought to be associated with the movements observed in seizures, but may be seen when the child is excited or emotional. Ataxia has also been noted in the population and may account for the wide-based, characteristic gait and some of the balance difficulties exhibited.

Speech-Language Issues

- Majority Nonverbal

- Augmentative and Alternative Communication

- Normal Hearing

- Oral-Motor Dysfunction

- Social Language

Oral Characteristics

In infancy, many children with Angelman syndrome develop feeding and swallowing difficulties. Poor sucking patterns can lead to poor weight gain, and it is not unheard of for these children to be diagnosed as "failure to thrive." Other oral behaviors noted in this population include mouthing, biting, drooling, chewing, rumination, and pica (an abnormal appetite for non-food items such as chalk or ashes).

Behaviors Related to Educational Planning

The terms *happy disposition, sociable,* and *loving* are often associated with Angelman syndrome. Frequent laughter, often inappropriate, has also been observed, though Alvares and Downing (1998) found only 50% of survey respondents scored the laughter of their children with Angelman syndrome as inappropriate. A short attention span and hyperactivity are seen as well as a natural inquisitiveness and the ability to become excited easily. Sleep disturbances are common. These children tend to love water and "rough and tumble" play rather than play involving concentration and attention. Other favorite items include noisy and musical toys, TV, and radio. Some stubbornness has also been observed.

Speech-Language Issues . . . .

The lack of expressive language development may be one of the most frustrating characteristics in children with Angelman syndrome, particularly for families with young children. The speech-language issues encountered in the population are explained in the following information.

Majority Nonverbal

The majority of children with Angelman syndrome are nonverbal, with the few verbal children having a very limited repertoire of words. Decreased babbling and cooing are described in their developmental histories.

Some of the severity of the expressive language disorder can be attributed to the level of mental retardation associated with the syndrome, though oral-motor dysfunction and lack of interaction opportunities may also inhibit expressive communication. A gap may exist between receptive and expressive language levels.

Augmentative and Alternative Communication

Since the majority of children with Angelman syndrome are nonverbal, alternative communication is a mode that deserves serious consideration. Beukelman and Mirenda (1998) present extensive information for making a decision concerning augmentative communication in their excellent textbook on the subject. Alvares and Downing (1998) list criteria to consider when selecting a communication modality for the child with Angelman syndrome, including the child's level of symbolic development, his motor and vision skills, his communicative partners, and the family's and client's preferences.

Gestures, signs, object boards or picture systems (low- or high-tech) may be appropriate augmentative modalities to consider for children with Angelman syndrome. The unique motor-movement patterns may interfere with certain signing forms (American Sign Language, Signing Exact English, etc.), but adapted signs within the motor abilities could be accepted. Impaired imitation abilities may also inhibit the learning of gesture and/or sign.

Normal Hearing

Hearing for children diagnosed with Angelman syndrome is reported to be within normal limits (Shprintzen, 1997). Other studies have reported the incidence of otitis media in the population, and the status of the middle ear should be monitored continually. The auditory channel may be a preferential modality for intervention purposes.

Oral-Motor Dysfunction

With a history of feeding difficulties, it is not surprising that children with Angelman syndrome often exhibit problems in the area of oral-motor functioning. The oral structure, with a wide mouth, irregularly-spaced teeth, prominent jaw, and tongue thrust, can also interfere with oral movement for speech. Imitation of oral-motor movements has been noted to be poor in these children, and drooling, mouthing, and biting have been observed.

Social Language

The child with Angelman syndrome is typically happy, sociable, and affectionate. This sociable nature and interest in others lays some foundation for observed pragmatic functions or intents noted in these children. Intents observed in nonverbal modes include instrumental (to get needs and wants met), regulatory (to regulate the behaviors of others), and interpersonal intents. Some joint attention and turn-taking skills are seen, but the child with Angelman syndrome does not generally initiate these interactions. Some limitations in the opportunity for a variety of social interactions have been thought to cause a decrease in pragmatic skills. The affectionate nature of this population also needs to be monitored as the children age to assure the pragmatic appropriateness of their nonverbal communication.

Intervention Issues . . . .

There is no known cure for Angelman syndrome, but early intervention and a team approach to treatment are beneficial. Major issues and goal areas to consider are summarized in the following information.

Augmentative and Alternative Communication

- Select a modality based on the individual child's needs and abilities.

- Sign to the child; an additional input mode may benefit the child's cognitive development.

- Investigate the possibility of using picture boards or electronic communicators.

- Select functional targets relative to the child's environment.

- Target contact gestures (close to the body or actual touch) prior to distal gestures (away from the body), such as pointing or hand gestures.

Oral Motor

- Attempt oral-motor exercises and movement patterns.

- Build oral imitation of vocal noises, especially those associated with pleasure, into turn-taking games.

- Decrease drooling, mouthing, and biting behaviors.

Social Language

- Increase eye contact.

- Increase the frequency of use for developed intents and functions of language.

- Increase the range of intent and function of language.

- Increase nonverbal and verbal turn-taking.

- Increase the number of turns per episode of interaction relating to one topic or event.

- Develop joint attention skills.

- Develop joint action skills.

Hyperactivity

- Use behavior-management techniques to reduce hyperactivity and increase attention. Use positive tangible and social reinforcers.

- Physical environmental planning with restricted areas of stimulation can benefit the child.

Task Analysis

- Breaking tasks down and teaching the sequence can assist the child in learning, particularly in the areas of self help and social skills.

Team Approach

- Use physical therapy to address gross-motor movement patterns, including the development of ambulation. Gait, weight-bearing issues, and joint mobility may also be addressed.

- Use occupational therapy to address sensory issues and fine-motor movements.

- An audiologist will assist in determining status of the middle ear.

- A nutritionist may be involved to assure these children get the nutritional intake required to gain weight early in life.

- Involve the family as primary caregivers for young members of this population.

Summary Comments · · · · · · · · · · · · · · · · ·

Angelman syndrome, the "happy puppet" syndrome, is a genetic neurological disorder with an incidence of one in 10,000 to one in 25,000 births. Developmental delays, particularly in the motor and communication domains, are among the most noted characteristics. A large, smiling mouth and prominent chin are common. Unusual movement patterns are exhibited, including hand flapping, fine tremors, and jerky limb movements. Poor feeding and swallowing in infancy is observed; many of these children are diagnosed as "failure to thrive" in their first few years. Oral behaviors such as mouthing, biting, drooling, and chewing continue as the child ages.

A large number of children with Angelman syndrome will remain nonverbal throughout their lives. With this in mind, augmentative and alternative communication strategies should be investigated for this population. Functional objectives set by a transdisciplinary team would be most beneficial.

References . . . .

Alvares, R. L. and Downing, S. F. "A Survey of Expressive Communication Skills in Children with Angelman Syndrome." *American Journal of Speech-Pathology*, Vol. 7, pp. 14-24, 1998.

Beukelman, M. *Augmentative and Alternative Communication: Management of Severe Communication Disorders, Second Edition.* Baltimore, MD: Brookes Publishing Co., 1998.

Miles, J. "Angelman Syndrome Information," 1997. [Online] Available: http://chem-faculty.ucsd.edu/harvey/asfsite/Web_Sites.html.

Shprintzen, R. J. *Genetics, Syndromes and Communication Disorders.* San Diego, CA: Singular Publishing Group, Inc., 1997.

Asperger's Syndrome

Characteristics

- Normal to above-average IQ and communication
- Significant pragmatic deficits
- Language differences
- Extreme interests and routines
- Motor, learning, and emotional problems

- egocentricity; poor social skills

- clumsiness

- usually diagnosed after age 24 months

- 1/1,000 to 1/7,000 live births; higher incidence for males than for females

- nonverbal learning disabilities

- rigidity

Syndrome Definition . . . .

Hans Asperger, an Austrian pediatrician, was the first to describe a population of children who had significant problems in social adjustment, clumsy movements, and extreme interests in bizarre subjects. While a specific cause was not known, Dr. Asperger theorized there was a genetic transmission of the disorder, noting a high incidence of similar characteristics in the fathers of the group of boys he was studying.

Dr. Asperger published his findings in 1944, almost at the same time that Dr. Leo Kanner labeled a group of individuals as "autistic." Dr. Kanner's definition of autism became well known, while Dr. Asperger's work wasn't carefully examined or circulated until Dr. Lorna Wing published a paper in 1981, noting close agreement of behavioral characteristics with those summarized by Asperger. Dr. Wing (cited in Attwood, 1998) listed the main characteristics of Asperger's syndrome as follows:

- lack of empathy
- naive, inappropriate, one-sided interaction
- little or no ability to form friendships

- pedantic, repetitive speech

- poor nonverbal communication

- intense absorption in certain subjects

- clumsy, poorly-coordinated movements and odd postures

Trevarthen et al. (1996) compiled a review of the primary features that major researchers agreed upon in diagnosing Asperger's syndrome. Their chart included the following:

- autistic social impairment

- clumsiness

- concrete or pedantic speech

- all-absorbing, circumscribed interests

- lack of appreciation for humor

- no significant delays in language or cognitive development

Asperger's syndrome is generally not recognized prior to 24 months of age. There is general agreement that Asperger's occurs more often in males than females. Incidence figures vary dramatically in the literature, ranging from one in every 1,000 to one in every 7,000 live births. A study in Sweden by Ehlers and Gilberg in 1993 (cited in Attwood, 1998) suggests an incidence for Asperger's syndrome as high as one in every 300 children.

Asperger's syndrome is recognized as a separate and distinct clinical entity from autism, but is included under the category of Pervasive Developmental Disorders and within the autistic spectrum of disabilities, as is Rett's syndrome. Note that Asperger's syndrome and high-functioning autism are NOT synonymous labels. Differences between the two can be identified, with the primary difference being that Asperger's syndrome characteristics are more consistent with right-hemisphere deficits, such as a nonverbal learning disability, while high-functioning autism characteristics are more consistent with left-hemisphere language/communication deficits (Trevarthen et al., 1996).

The diagnostic criteria for differential diagnosis of Asperger's syndrome are included in the *Diagnostic and Statistical Manual of Mental Disorders, Fourth Edition* (1994) and are compatible with the *World Health Organization's International Classification of Diseases, Tenth Edition*. Asperger's syndrome is included on Axis I, Clinical Disorders diagnosed during infancy, childhood, or early adolescence. The accepted medical diagnostic criteria from *DSM-IV* are summarized in the chart on the following page.

Asperger's Syndrome

- Significant impairment in social interaction
- Restricted, repetitive, and stereotyped patterns of behavior, interests, or activities
- Significant impairment in social, occupational, or other areas of functioning
- Generally age-appropriate development in language, cognitive development, self-help skills, adaptive behavior (except for social interaction), and environmental curiosity

Behavioral Characteristics Profile . . . .

Behavioral characteristics presented by various experts were listed in the previous section. The following section consolidates the authors' opinions and expands the explanation of how these characteristics would be observed by practicing professionals.

Normal to Above-Average IQ and Communication Development

Most individuals with Asperger's syndrome demonstrate normal intelligence; mental retardation is not typically associated with the syndrome. That does not mean that formal intelligence testing attempted during early years of intervention will necessarily yield results within one standard deviation of the norm (IQ at or above 70). Assessment is completed through communication and social interaction. Before intense intervention efforts are initiated, a child will rarely relate to a stranger well enough to reflect his cognitive potential accurately in a testing situation. Informal observation will be required to supplement standardized performance measures during the first several years of education. However, an individual with Asperger's syndrome should eventually demonstrate performance on formal IQ assessment that reflects cognitive capabilities within a normal range.

Development of fundamental speech-language skills is also relatively normal. In fact, many children with Asperger's syndrome are somewhat precocious in acquiring the ability to talk. Concrete, factual information is often absorbed and repeated in a monotone manner. Basic sentence structure and phonology (i.e., phonemes of the language) develop early and without extensive remediation. Difficulties begin to appear as language becomes more abstract, interactive, and social in nature.

Significant Pragmatic Deficits

The ability to interact socially is significantly impaired within Asperger's syndrome. The difference in Asperger's versus autism can be discriminated in the area of social behavior. The child with autism is aloof, withdrawn, and fairly oblivious to social interaction. The child with Asperger's syndrome has an interest in other people socially, but suffers from a definite lack of social-interaction skills. Peer interaction is significantly discrepant within Asperger's syndrome. These children usually favor interacting with older or younger individuals. Adults are preferred for social interaction because adults are more tolerant of social differences, more interesting, and more knowledgeable about carrying on a conversation. Play is often preferred with much younger children because the demands to follow social rules are less strenuous than with peers.

Individuals with Asperger's syndrome have extreme difficulty learning and responding to social cues. Verbal comments that are tolerated from a young child who might not know better become problematic as the child becomes older. Behavior in social situations is often perceived as rude or embarrassing to other people, while the individual with Asperger's syndrome is oblivious to any problems. The child with Asperger's syndrome does not process social cues or notice subtle suggestions.

The inability to perceive the needs and desires of others is also part of the social deficits of Asperger's syndrome. A lack of empathy for the feelings or situations of other people can significantly compromise the appropriateness of responses from an individual with Asperger's syndrome. While the children are generally affectionate with parents and siblings, their emotional reactions tend to be driven by their own needs rather than in response to family members' needs. This egocentric focus makes it difficult to relate to others and empathize with them.

Language Differences

Language comprehension is often rather superficial and concrete within Asperger's syndrome. These children do fairly well with basic receptive language knowledge, but begin to experience difficulty with abstract concepts. Their interpretations are often literal for colloquial language and idiomatic expressions used daily in the home and school settings. Children with Asperger's syndrome can completely miss implied meanings.

Expressive language problems are often a result of the lack of social awareness and empathetic responses. Vocal production is often mono-tone, robotic, and artificial sounding. Language patterns can be rather formal in structure and pedantic or self-righteous in tone. Verbalizations are often absent of accompanying facial expression or gestures. Body language can be stiff or peculiar and sometimes seems to contradict content being expressed.

Extreme Interests and Routines

A common feature cited repeatedly in regard to Asperger's syndrome is a total self-absorption in specific interests. Children can perseverate extensively on obscure or unusual topics of interest to the exclusion of everything else. These fetishes lead to a certain eccentricity associated with the disorder. For example, some children can identify every teacher in the school by the car models they drive.

An extreme reliance on routines is also very characteristic of Asperger's syndrome. Families and teachers often relay stories of how a certain task has to be completed exactly the same way or these children will become very distressed. Perfectionistic tendencies are also noted. Some of these children cannot stand to make a mistake when writing their names and will erase until there are holes in the paper. Sometimes these children refuse to participate in class for fear of getting an answer wrong. Rituals and routines are one way of alleviating some of the stress within various settings to insure a task is done the right way.

Motor-Coordination Problems

An interesting feature of Asperger's syndrome that differentiates it from autism is clumsiness. While deficits in motor development are typical in autism, gross-motor clumsiness is cited within Asperger's. Children develop basic motor skills for self-help tasks, but are not particularly adept or skilled in motor movement. This inconsistency can be seen in odd postures and movement patterns in children with Asperger's syndrome.

Significant problems in fine-motor coordination are also typical in Asperger's syndrome, especially with graphic skills. Many children with the syndrome never develop neat or legible handwriting. Pencil grip is tense and pressure is very hard, resulting frequently in torn paper. Letters are large and visual perception for spacing on the page is poor. Fine-motor compensation is necessary through use of a computer or laptop to alleviate frustration and reduce time required for written responses.

Learning Problems

The learning profile within Asperger's syndrome is similar to a nonverbal learning disability. Right-hemisphere skills are usually cited as the primary aspects interfering with learning. Verbal language skills are strong for concrete functional information, but significantly impaired for interpreting humor, nuance, and subtle nonverbal cues. Problems in visual integration are consistent with this profile of learning difficulties and cited in conjunction with Asperger's syndrome. In addition, organization skills can be very poor despite the presence of rituals and routines. These children often complete tasks with no concept of time, working very slowly and ignoring or not understanding deadlines and due dates for projects or assignments. A child might not follow a teacher's directions because the child doesn't realize an implied time frame of immediate compliance.

Children with Asperger's syndrome often demonstrate a keen fascination with letters and numbers at an early age. Hyperlexia, a precocious ability to decode the sound-symbol system for oral reading, can be a common feature of the learning profile within Asperger's syndrome. While oral reading is advanced, the ability to comprehend and process content read is significantly impaired.

Mental rigidity is another aspect of this lack of processing (i.e., attaching meaning to stimuli) that occurs frequently in Asperger's syndrome. Thinking patterns can be very rigid. Concepts are viewed as black or white, with subtle variations almost impossible for them to understand. For example, a specific number can be "few" in some situations but "many" in another situation; it is all relative. That way of interpreting information is extremely challenging to individuals with Asperger's syndrome. The egocentric components also contribute to mental rigidity; they tend to see situations from their perspective only. Rules and laws can be very difficult to explain to children who only see it from their own perspectives.

Emotional Problems

Children with Asperger's syndrome typically have a normal to high IQ paired with awareness and interest in the world, but they have poor skills to cope. This impairment can create secondary emotional problems for individuals with Asperger's syndrome. At an early intervention level, an understanding of this possibility is important for the professional involved in remedial efforts to monitor frustration and insure positive experiences.

Depression is the primary emotional problem cited with Asperger's syndrome. Obsessive-compulsive disorder and anxiety/panic attacks are also natural outgrowths from the ritualistic, perfectionistic characteristics of the syndrome. It is not unusual to begin anti-anxiety medication around the onset of puberty to help a child cope with the overwhelming and confusing stimuli of the world.

Speech-Language Issues . . . .

Areas of concern to the speech-language pathologist dealing with Asperger's syndrome result primarily from the extreme social deficits and lack of awareness for social cues. Other issues are related to processing stimuli accurately, usually compromised by egocentric focus and mental rigidity or concreteness. Issues in the area of speech-language are discussed in the following information.

Pragmatic Language

Understanding social messages and rules is a subtle skill that is extremely weak in Asperger's syndrome. A child doesn't often pay attention to social cues, such as an adult lowering her speaking volume in church or a movie theatre to suggest that a child talk more softly. Violating social rules, such as commenting on or asking about something inappropriate in public, embarrasses teachers and parents, but doesn't usually disturb the child with

Asperger's syndrome. This subtle aspect of language must be addressed very directly. Don't assume anything; explain everything.

In conjunction with learning to understand social rules and cues, it is important to specifically teach appropriate social behavior. Children with Asperger's syndrome can be unjustly disciplined in an educational setting for behavioral violations that a teacher assumed the child understood. Because these children have normal intelligence and verbal communication skills, professionals tend to overestimate their understanding and development of social manners. Social skills should be directly taught through demonstration, role play, and daily routine practice.

Receptive Language

The fascination with letters and numbers can lead a professional to unfair assumptions regarding interpretation of meaning from information recited or read by a child with Asperger's syndrome.

The ability to accurately attach meaning to stimuli (i.e., processing) and insure pictures or images in the brain cannot be inferred or assumed; the reality must always be checked through questions. Specific interests for which a child with Asperger's syndrome can recite myriads of data does not insure that simple functional aspects are understood within the facts.

Comprehension of figurative language is also challenging to the child with Asperger's syndrome. The child who demonstrates an excellent memory for facts of interest may hear an adult say "an elephant never forgets" and have no idea what that means. Colloquial uses of figurative language incorporated into classroom directions can be especially problematic. For example, *Hang onto your seats, Line up on the wall,* and *Just throw it on my desk* can create problems if interpreted literally. Humor, sarcasm, and idiomatic expressions that surround us every day can cause great anxiety and misunderstanding for the child with Asperger's syndrome.

Expressive Language

Vocal characteristics can be very different in children with Asperger's syndrome. Vocalizations may sound rather flat, due to monotone, robotic phrasing and inflection patterns. Some children sound like small adults when stating their opinion, and their authoritative manner isn't always appreciated by teachers, even though no offense is intended.

Nonverbal aspects of communication can be significantly different in Asperger's syndrome. Eye gaze, posture, facial expression, and gestures may be exaggerated, completely absent, or may appear to contradict verbal content.

Discourse

Conversational rules are typically poorly understood by individuals with Asperger's syndrome. Children will often rudely interrupt, not understanding the social rules governing when or how to gain entrance to a conversation in a polite manner. It is not uncommon for a child with Asperger's disorder to suddenly switch topic to an area of her interest or fetish, ignoring other conversational cues. Using small talk to initiate or terminate conversation is also extremely difficult for these children, and usually poorly executed.

Intervention Issues . . . .

Focus on building social skills during initial remediation efforts for Asperger's syndrome. Children with this disability have excellent potential for regular education placement and progress when early intervention helps to develop the social skills that allow them to function productively in a classroom setting. Professionals should be careful not to make assumptions based on a level of skills demonstrated in some areas, such as hyperlexia. Inconsistencies in language should be targeted directly to insure comprehension and alleviate the child's frustration. Primary goals for intervention are summarized below.

Social Skills Training

- Understanding the reasons for social rules should be taught directly. Carol Gray has devised a series of Social Stories to use with children who don't understand the subtle rules that govern our everyday lives. The stories have an established formula and are read

Intervention Issues

- Social Skills Training

- Vocal Inflection and Prosody

- Receptive Language Comprehension

- Conversational Skills

- Team Approach

to the children over several days to concretely and directly teach the reasons for certain behavioral expectations.

- The ability to read social cues should also be directly targeted. Non-verbal body language is a good place to start. Use a mirror and have children focus on your face to read emotions, such as *happy, sad, angry,* or *in a hurry.* Discuss the facial expression and body posture that sends that message. Develop visual and or verbal cards to discriminate meaning. For example, "The teacher keeps looking at her watch. What is the nonverbal social message?"

- Establish routines and rituals to practice sending appropriate social cues. Again, create visual/verbal cards with messages to send. The child and teacher can take turns sending and guessing the social message.

- Appropriate social interaction with peers should also be taught directly. Begin through demonstration and role play as adult and child. Once the child has demonstrated competence in various social situations with an adult, invite a peer to join. For example, the professional might teach the game of Go Fish and incorporate social manners for turn taking, making requests, etc. Once the child has mastered the social behavior to play with the adult, invite a peer to join the game. Gradually add more peers and fade the adult to monitor the social situation but not actually be involved.

Vocal Inflection and Prosody

- Children's stories can be told and re-enacted with various character voice changes to provide practice in rate, volume, inflection, etc. For example, *The Three Bears* allows a child to play with various pitch and volume levels when reciting lines for the papa, mama, and baby bears. Using children's literature removes the stress of trying to generate the language and vocal characteristics. The teacher's model can be imitated to focus the child's energy primarily on practicing vocal changes rather than cognitive challenges.

- Modeling can very directly target specific vocal characteristics of concern. For example, a child who is extremely monotone can be asked to play Simon Says and copy the clinician's vocal model. Rate, rhythm, pitch, inflection, and volume are all possible specific modeling targets.

- Automatic speech can be very effective for targeting practice on vocal production aspects. Songs, rhymes, finger plays, etc., are excellent preschool techniques to target exploration of vocal aspects.

- Use creative drama and video-taping to motivate and allow the child to objectively view his vocal production after producing it. One effective strategy is to have the child pretend to be a news broadcaster or TV/ movie star. Videotape the child presenting a short message to the camera. Then view the tape together, discussing volume, inflection, or other targeted vocal characteristics.

Receptive Language Comprehension

- Target the ability to accurately process verbal information directly, beginning at a very concrete level and progressing into abstract concepts, such as the fifty Boehm concepts. Begin by addressing conceptual language goals related to functional situations in the child's home and school settings.

- Incorporate reality checks on reading comprehension through consistent questions. The child may become upset by the interruptions, but you cannot otherwise assume the child has perceived and understood what she reads. Use visual prompts whenever possible to avoid the child's factual repetition of non-meaningful verbalization.

- Children with high IQ within Asperger's syndrome enjoy the challenge of verbal language. Humor, idiomatic expressions, similes, colloquialisms, and similar language nuances can present a stimulating and motivating challenge to the child. One preschool child with Asperger's syndrome used to come to the therapy session and ask to work on "multiple meanings or idiomatic expressions"! This goal may be too high level for many preschool children, but choose targets specific to everyday, functional situations appropriate for each child.

Conversation Skills

- Teach aspects of verbal discourse (e.g., topic initiation, maintenance, and termination; conversational turn-taking; interruptions) through identification of various features by observing videos, other children, or adults engaged in conversation. Identify one focus to target at a time. For example, "Today we'll look for how people end a conversation or let other people know they are finished talking."

- Teach nonverbal aspects of conversation (e.g., eye gaze, facial expression, gestures) by identifying a targeted objective as you watch videos or other people engaged in conversation. Turn down the sound and focus the child on only face, gesture, body movements, etc.

- Practice targeted aspects by allowing the child to use role play and rituals to develop confidence with conversation skills. Rehearse typical social situations (such as going to the dentist) by using puppets, mirrors, re-enacting events, and role play in the therapy setting before initiating carryover to the real world.

- Carryover of practiced conversational skills in real life situations is critical if the child with Asperger's syndrome is to achieve control of his anxiety to implement the skills taught in therapy.

Team Approach

- Occupational therapy may be addressing sensory issues. Exploring compensatory strategies for fine-motor graphic skills is important, even though handwriting can be directly targeted.

- Physical therapy may suggest strategies to improve gross-motor coordination.

- Address uneven learning patterns with a learning disabilities teacher. Appropriate compensatory strategies will alleviate frustration with academic tasks. Routines and rituals are important to control anxiety and perfectionistic, obsessive-compulsive tendencies.

- In-service will be necessary with regular education teachers to make sure they understand the nuances of the disability and have realistic expectations for the child.

- A psychologist may need to monitor emotional stability and provide counseling services as needed if the child becomes overwhelmed or frustrated in the educational setting.

- A need for medication is likely at some point, although not during early years of school. Consider coordination with a pediatrician or a medical professional.

Summary Comments . . . .

Asperger's syndrome is a fascinating disorder. The children diagnosed with this disorder are generally memorable, delightful, and challenging. While relatively new as a diagnostic label (since 1981 when Dr. Wing publicized Dr. Asperger's information), the incidence may be much higher than previously thought. Numerous individuals who found their niches in life might have actually had Asperger's syndrome, but it was never diagnosed. Their peculiar, eccentric ways were tolerated because of their normal IQ and the contributions they had made in highly specialized areas.

Temple Grandin includes a chapter on the idea of genius in her book *Thinking in Pictures*. In it, she makes a case for such scientists as Einstein possibly having Asperger's disorder due to his poor social skills and lack of developed social behavior. One family, when receiving a diagnosis of Asperger's syndrome for their four-year-old daughter, also received the same diagnosis for the father! He was a college professor in art, and his poor social skills were considered part of an artistic temperament and, therefore, accepted.

One picture to use to conceptualize Asperger's syndrome is the android Data from *Star Trek: The Next Generation*. Data is a walking encyclopedia of knowledge, but has great difficulty knowing when too much information is being presented. He struggles to accurately read social cues and is puzzled by nonliteral use of language. Emotions are alien to him, but fascinating and frustrating. He studies human beings to try to better understand and participate in the strange social rituals required. Many children with Asperger's syndrome face the same challenges on a daily basis and are perceived in much the same way as Data is by his fellow crewmates.

Asperger's syndrome has a very positive prognosis when social skills are addressed and a child's acute interests can be channeled. With intense, focused early intervention, the excellent potential of children with Asperger's syndrome is beginning to be realized in the educational setting. Normal and gifted programs are benefitting from the unique insight these individuals bring to an educational setting, once language and learning difficulties are understood, acknowledged as legitimate, and compensated for appropriately.

References . . . .

American Psychiatric Association. *Diagnostic and Statistical Manual of Mental Disorders, Fourth Edition.* Washington, D.C.: American Psychiatric Association, 1994.

Attwood, T. *Asperger's Syndrome: A Guide for Parents and Professionals.* London, England: Jessica Kingsley Publishers, 1998.

Frith, U. *Autism and Asperger Syndrome.* Cambridge, England: Cambridge University Press, 1991.

Gilbert, P. *The A-Z Reference Book of Syndromes and Inherited Disorders, Second Edition.* London, England: Chapman & Hall, 1996.

Grandin, T. *Thinking in Pictures and Other Reports from My Life with Autism.* New York, NY: Doubleday, 1995.

Gray, C. *The New Social Story Book.* Arlington, TX: Future Horizons, Inc., 1994.

Powers, M. "Diagnosis of Autism and Related Pervasive Developmental Disorders." Eastern Illinois University Summer Institute on Autism, 1998.

Trevarthen, C., Aitken, K., Papoudi, D., and Robarts, J. *Children with Autism: Diagnosis and Interventions to Meet Their Needs.* London, England: Jessica Kingsley Publishers, 1996.

Autism

Characteristics

- Problems in reciprocal social interaction
- Delays and differences in communication
- Stereotypic behaviors with objects and the environment
- Abnormal responses to sensory stimulation
- Mental retardation; mental rigidity

- physical, neurological brain disorder

- 15/10,000 live births

- higher incidence for males

- continuum of severity from mild to severe

- lifelong disability

- impaired speech and language functioning

Syndrome Definition . . . .

Autism means "self," and the term was introduced in 1943 by Dr. Leo Kanner to describe a population of isolated individuals who failed to relate to other people and the environment. While not titled as such, autism is a syndrome disorder defined by multiple characteristics to result in a diagnosis. Neither a definitive cause nor a medical evaluation for diagnosis is available yet, although certain trends are beginning to emerge from the research. One example is the increased risk of autism within families, acknowledging the genetic link in many cases.

Autism is a physical neurological disorder of the brain that occurs on a continuum of severity from mild to severe. It has been cited in all ethnic backgrounds around the world. The incidence figures currently cited are usually about 15 per 10,000 births. Males are affected more frequently than females, ranging from 2.5 to 4 males to one female. It is noted to be the third most common developmental disability, with only mental retardation and cerebral palsy occurring more frequently. Despite reports in popular literature, autism is a lifelong disability that is not cured but responds well to intervention efforts to modify components of the disorder.

Autism is included within the category of Pervasive Developmental Disorders (PDD), which indicates pervasive and significant deficits across several developmental areas. Autism needs to be differentiated from other Pervasive Developmental Disorders of Rett's, Asperger's, and Childhood Disintegrative. The following chart summarizes diagnostic features of Autism according to the *Diagnostic and Statistical Manual of Mental Disorders, Fourth Edition.*

Autistic Disorder

- Impairment in social interaction

- Impairments in communication

- Restricted, repetitive, and stereotyped patterns of behavior, interests, and activities

- Delays or abnormal functioning with onset prior to three years of age

---

Autism is also part of the *Individuals with Disabilities Act (IDEA),* which by federal law designates autism as a primary disability within special education. This educational label allows special services to be provided in the school setting for all of the syndrome features. Each state delineates its own interpretation of the criterion for diagnosing autism from the specifications listed in *IDEA.* A portion of the federal definition follows:

> *Autism* means a developmental disability significantly affecting verbal and nonverbal communication and social interaction, generally evident before age three, that adversely affects the child's educational performance.

Other characteristics often associated with autism include the following:
- engagement in repetitive activities and stereotyped movements
- resistance to environmental change or change in daily routines
- unusual response to sensory experiences

Autism can co-occur with other major disabilities, such as blindness, deafness, cerebral palsy, and Down syndrome. Besides the primary diagnostic characteristics listed in the *DSM-IV,* additional components are possible within the syndrome profile, such as hyperlexia and fine- and gross-motor deficits. Mental retardation is noted to occur in 75% of the individuals with autism, but those estimates are based on diagnosis prior to publication of the *DSM-IV,* which did not accommodate diagnosis in the milder end of the autistic spectrum. Despite variability in severity, the most dominant feature in all individuals with autism is the aloof, isolated characteristic of minimal awareness to social interaction physically, facially, and communicatively.

Behavioral Characteristics Profile . . . .

Autism is a developmental disorder that is diagnosed from the behavioral characteristics evidenced. Careful observation usually yields the syndrome profile within a relatively short period of time if the observation occurs in a natural or comfortable setting for the child. For diagnosis, the characteristics observed should be organized to determine if the observed components meet diagnostic criteria.

While the autistic syndrome can have a large variety of characteristic features, the main high-frequency behavioral characteristics that constitute the profile associated with autism are summarized in the following information.

Problems in Reciprocal Social Interaction

The inability to relate to other people in a social context is one of the most striking features of autism. Children can appear oblivious to social cues and people. Eye contact can be extremely limited, if occurring at all. Children seem to have an internal focus and fail to respond to external stimuli, unless of their own choice. Even when an adult points out or requests a social mannerism, the child may appear confused or unaware of what the adult is talking about. There is a definite social naivete for interaction with other people. Children might also resist social interaction by circling the perimeter of the environment to avoid coming in contact with other people.

Delays and Differences in Communication

Speech and language development is always impaired to some extent within autism. While some areas follow a normal developmental progression (such as phonological acquisition in a verbal child), other areas are very aberrant. Therefore, you see both delays and differences in communication developmental patterns.

Echolalic speech (repeating speech previously heard) is very typical within autism. Children often repeat what they hear, much like a parrot, but without comprehending the language content. While imitation is a normal stage of language development, it is evidenced to an extreme degree within autism. Children also memorize language and songs, such as commercials and sayings, and repetitively reproduce them without understanding the meaning. For this reason, expressive language may develop through this echoed practice effect, exceeding actual receptive comprehension. It is not unusual to have higher expressive language scores than receptive for children who have autism.

Literature on autism suggests that approximately 40% of individuals with autism are mute, with little or no useable verbal communication. This phenomena is probably due to apraxia as part of the neurological profile of the syndrome. These children are not choosing to withhold verbal communication as once hypothesized, but are unable to voluntarily program the neurological systems controlling the speech mechanism.

Other speech abnormalities associated with autism include a lack of vocal inflection, resulting in very flat, monotone verbal production. Jargon and original language terms are also noted, along with echolalia. Volume, rate, and prosodic differences are frequent and can be extreme enough to significantly impair intelligibility. Speech production can sound very robotic and artificial.

Stereotypic Behaviors

Children with autism become very threatened and confused when leaving their internal world to process external stimuli. A vehicle for coping with the stress of unknown external demands is to rely on routines or sameness when facing the world. Children resist changes in schedule, furniture arrangement, driving routes, clothing, etc. Play patterns can also be ritualistic; these children may play with the same toy in the same place in the same way each day unless interrupted or patterned to do otherwise. The behavioral components of autism are often the most confusing and disturbing for parents and professionals to deal with.

Self-stimulatory movements are rhythmic, repetitive motor patterns in which the child engages. Examples typically seen within autism are hand flapping, rocking, rubbing, chewing, humming, and spinning. The perseverative movement patterns seem to be comforting or calming for the child but can be disruptive to other individuals in the environment.

Fixation on certain topics or activities is also typical of autism. Children may be fascinated by trains, types of shoes, or certain insects. It is often hard to intrude and break a child out of a perseverative interest.

Speech-Language Issues

- Semantic Language

- Receptive Language

- Expressive Language

- Pragmatic Language

- General Educational Concerns

Abnormal Responses to Sensory Stimulation

The physical nature of autism appears to have a bio-chemical aspect which results in hyper-responsive and hypo-responsive reactions to stimuli. Hypersensitivity to smell, taste, and texture in the oral cavity accounts for the large number of children with extremely selective eating patterns. Overly sensitive responses to auditory stimuli are also frequently observed, as evidenced by children with autism who keep their fingers in their ears to block out sound. Direct visual contact can be overwhelming, resulting in a slightly off-center eye gaze for visual stimuli.

Mental Retardation; Mental Rigidity

Impairment in cognitive functioning of varying degrees of severity is well documented within the syndrome of autism. The more severe the mental retardation, the worse the prognosis for success in intervention efforts to modify the behavioral characteristics of the disorder. Even when IQ appears to be within a normal range, challenges to learning still exist. Children with autism have difficulty processing abstract information, only understanding more concrete, clear, and functional information. These children can demonstrate remarkable recall and memorization skills, but their functional application is often lacking. For example, a child may be able to calculate numbers quickly without understanding the value of the numerical result.

Speech-Language Issues . . . .

The area of speech-language is the largest deficit area within autism. Pragmatic language is the ability to communicate in varying social contexts and is the first diagnostic feature in the *DSM-IV* criteria. The second criterion is in relation to communication. In total, it could be argued that speech-language accounts for two-thirds of the disorder features (since the fourth criterion is onset age). Therefore, a speech-language pathologist is a critical professional in achieving accurate diagnosis and intervention within autism. The issues of concern are global and diverse in relation to communication, making the task of deciding where to start intervention almost overwhelming at times. Significant issues are summarized in the following information.

Semantic Language

Receptive language comprehension can be significantly impaired within autism, but occurs on a continuum of severity. Children with autism have difficulty attaching meaning to auditory stimuli. Many don't understand that a message is encoded in the sound patterns swirling around them in the environment. Concrete object vocabulary can develop fairly well, but more abstract language presents challenges. Literal versus figurative interpretation of language expressions is fairly common. It is important to supplement verbal language with visual stimuli and physical demonstration to insure accurate interpretation of meaning. Many of our language terms change meaning, based on the context in which they are used. This flexibility also presents problems for the child with autism. Higher levels of semantic language knowledge, such as verbal reasoning, problem solving, idioms, analogies, etc., are difficult to establish for the child with autism.

Expressive language issues cover a wide range. The primary challenge centers on establishing intelligible, meaningful verbal output. Many children with autism demonstrate idiosyncratic language patterns and struggle to adapt to our language system. Apraxia contributes to mutism in just under half of the individuals with autism. Non-meaningful echoed speech occurs with high frequency, interfering with meaningful output. Vocal production patterns can also be deviant, ranging from monotone, robotic speech to very exaggerated, sing-songy verbal patterns. Non-verbal attributes that serve to enhance speech, such as eye contact, gestures, and facial expression, are often absent.

Pragmatic Language

The ability to understand and modify communication within social situations is a subtle aspect of language that is significantly impaired within children who have autism. The language problems create difficulty for the child in attempting to process or attach meaning to the actual words spoken. It becomes almost impossible for the child to also pay attention to facial expression, gestures, and vocal inflection to scaffold additional meaning on the words. In addition, the child with autism seems fairly oblivious to social cues from others, due to the self-centered nature of the disorder; it is extremely difficult for the child to understand a situation from the perspective of another person. Immediate self-gratification is often the only focus of preschool children, resulting in social interactive challenges within the educational setting.

General Educational Concerns

Behavior problems are usually the first educational concern and a striking feature of autism. Ritualistic behaviors, rigid insistence on sameness, unusual attachments to certain objects, self-stimulatory movements, and obsessive routines are extremely confounding and significantly interfere with learning. Tantrums can be triggered with little or no apparent warning, significantly disrupting the learning environment for other children.

Mental rigidity contributes to some unique learning patterns and challenges. Children with autism can often recall or reproduce minute, detailed information, but be unable to answer simple questions about the content recited. Reading comprehension can be very poor, despite excellent oral reading skills. Math calculations might be quite easy, but story/word math problems are impossible. An unevenness in learning patterns across subjects is fairly typical within the disorder of autism. Mental retardation occurs in the majority of individuals with autism, further compromising learning potential.

Intervention Issues . . . .

The speech-language pathologist is a key professional in intervention efforts for autism. While communication deficits account for the majority of disorder features, adjunct professionals involved with the child are important in stimulating language development in conjunction with the speech-pathologist. For therapy to be effective, services must be functional and integrated with real-life situations. A structured, consistent approach will be most effective for facilitating learning. Incorporate motor-movement opportunities on a regular basis to enhance attention and minimize behavioral disruptions. The following information summarizes the primary goals the speech-language pathologist needs to address within the syndrome of autism.

Intervention Issues

- Conceptual Receptive Language Comprehension and Processing

- Expressive Language Production

- Pragmatic Language Development

- Team Approach

Conceptual Receptive Language Comprehension and Processing

- Evaluate language comprehension continually in everyday situations through questions and picture/object confrontation to insure understanding.

- Introduce conceptual vocabulary items (e.g., Boehm basic concepts) in functional experiences that have a concrete impact on the child.

- Provide multimodality (e.g., use of visual, tactile, verbal stimulation) demonstration and assistance to clarify meaning while minimizing your verbal input.

- Use gestures and signs to supplement verbal input to clarify and improve the opportunity for the child to attach meaning and understand information presented.

- Simplify your verbal language, using telegraphic speech to facilitate comprehension.

Expressive Language Production

- If the child is nonverbal, initiate oral-motor exercises to stimulate neurological development of the speech mechanism. Begin at respiration to establish a controlled and sustained airflow (whistles, candles, bubbles, party favors, horns, etc). Work toward voicing (kazoos, humming) and into resonance and articulation.

- Use songs, poems, fingerplays, etc., to promote automatic speech production.

- Explore and develop alternative augmentative forms of communication based on cognitive level of performance and apraxic severity.

- Gradually shape echolalia from non-meaningful output to meaningful. Don't try to extinguish echolalic speech unless it is extremely perseverative and non-meaningful.

- Monitor and address speech production aspects as necessary. A monotone pattern of voice production could be targeted through exploration of vocal inflection through retelling children's stories with characters of varying pitches and intensity (e.g., *The Three Bears* or *Three Billy Goats Gruff*). Use exaggerated inflection to encourage imitation of vocal variety from your model.

Pragmatic Language Development

- Develop both verbal and nonverbal turn-taking skills. Engage in an activity, such as putting a puzzle together where the pieces are shared. Look at a book together and alternate who turns the page.

- Develop an awareness of social rules through explanation, stories, and examples to help a child understand the reason behind social customs. Carol Gray's Social Stories are an excellent resource in this area.

- Develop daily routines that incorporate social manners, such as saying *please* and *thank you* at snack time and *hello* and *good-bye* when entering and leaving the classroom.

- Practice beginning rules of discourse, such as not interrupting other people who are talking, and what to say to initiate or end conversation. Teach a child how to ask to use a toy, go to the bathroom, move a child out of his or her space, etc.

- Teach and practice in a mirror the development of nonverbal aspects to support communication, such as eye contact when initiating verbal communication, facial expression to indicate emotions, body posture and positioning, etc.

Team Approach

- The teacher will need to understand how to balance movement activities with sitting. Allow down time for the child on a regular basis to calm and cope with environmental stimuli, and limit stimuli to focus the child's attention to task.

- A behavioral consultant might be necessary to program management strategies and ideas to modify disruptive or self-abusive behaviors.

- A psychologist should document the child's nonverbal cognitive performance level for assistance in educational programming. Circumventing verbal demands as well as minimizing social communicative responses in testing will yield more accurate results of actual cognitive potential.

- An occupational therapist may be involved to evaluate and program for fine-motor deficits that impact handwriting and visual-spatial skills. Sensory hyper and hypo responses can also be evaluated and programmed for with consultation from the occupational therapist.

- Physical therapy may be involved to evaluate and program for gross-motor deficits.

- Music therapy can program to desensitize hypersensitive hearing as well as to relax and calm a child who has become overwhelmed in the educational setting.

- Involve a physician to monitor medication, eating habits, and general health and nutrition.

Summary Comments . . . .

Autism is a fascinating, complex syndrome disorder that occurs on a continuum of severity. Although it was identified in the 1940's, many misconceptions continue to exist in regard to the disability, sometimes preventing accurate diagnosis and intervention. While the incidence of autism has steadily increased over the last decade, prognosis has also significantly improved with early identification and initiation of intervention efforts. The increase in incidence has raised the public profile of autism, and research efforts are being concentrated in an attempt to understand and better diagnose and treat the syndrome.

Stories of cures and remarkable changes due to various treatments abound in popular reading sources, but autism is a lifelong disability that does not go away. However, the symptoms respond well to intensive early intervention efforts, and modification can significantly mask the features over time. A critical feature impacting prognosis is the adjunct characteristic of mental retardation. If mental retardation is absent in the autistic profile, the possibility of independent functioning in the future is enhanced. If severe mental retardation is present, the cognitive impairment further compromises prognosis.

Many features associated with autism, such as self-stimulatory movements, also occur in other disabilities. This fact has led to an over-identification of the syndrome in some cases, as well as confusion in what the disorder actually is. Strict adherence to the diagnostic criteria of multiple features, consistent with syndrome diagnosis, is important to differentiate autism from other associated deficits.

The multifaceted nature of this disorder necessitates the involvement of multiple professionals in the treatment process. Services must be coordinated and integrated to maximize effectiveness.

●　　　　●　　　　●　　　　●　　　　●　　　　●　　　　●

References . . . .

American Psychiatric Association. *Diagnostic and Statistical Manual of Mental Disorders, Fourth Edition.* Washington, D.C.: American Psychiatric Association, 1994.

Batshaw, M. and Perret, Y. *Children with Disabilities: A Medical Primer, Third Edition.* Baltimore, MD: Paul H. Brookes Publishing Co., 1992.

Gerlach, E. *Autism Treatment Guide.* Eugene, OR: Four Leaf Press, 1993.

Grandin, T. *Thinking in Pictures and Other Reports from My Life with Autism.* New York, NY: Doubleday, 1995.

Gray, C. *The New Social Story Book.* Arlington, TX: Future Horizons, Inc., 1994.

Powers, M. *Children with Autism: A Parent's Guide.* Rockville, MD: Woodbine House, 1989.

Richard, G. *The Source for Autism.* East Moline, IL: LinguiSystems, Inc., 1997.

● ● ● ● ● ● ● ●

Down Syndrome

Characteristics

- Mental retardation
- Health issues
- Physical characteristics
- Facial features

Syndrome Definition . . . .

- leading genetic cause of mental retardation

- 1/700-800 live births

- equal numbers of males and females

- hearing loss

- voice disorders

- articulation disorders

Down syndrome is a constellation of symptoms with a common genetic cause. Down syndrome was first described by Dr. John Langdon Down in 1866 in a paper including a complete physical description of the condition. The genetic cause for Down syndrome was identified in 1959, with trisomy of chromosome 21 being pinpointed. Two other genetic mechanisms involving chromosome 21, translocation and mosaicism, can also cause Down syndrome.

Down syndrome is considered one of the most common chromosomal disorders with incidences reported at one in 700/800 live births (Miller et al., 1998; Mervis et al., 1998; Jung, 1989). A clinical diagnosis based on a pattern of recognizable characteristics is common, and a chromosomal analysis should be performed on any child suspected of having Down syndrome to verify the diagnosis.

Down syndrome is the leading genetic cause of mental retardation, and specific medical problems are seen. Increased risk of abnormalities in almost every organ system is reported by Batshaw, 1997. Males and females are equally affected by Down syndrome, and the incidence increases with maternal and paternal age. There has been a decrease in prevalence since the onset of prenatal diagnosis, and genetic counseling for future pregnancies is available. In 96 percent of cases, the cause is an accidental change in chromosome 21 and is not inherited (Miller & Leddy, 1998). The trisomy of chromosome 21 causes physical malformations more often as a result of incomplete development rather than deviant development in utero.

Behavioral Characteristics Profile . . . .

The primary behavioral characteristics of children with Down syndrome are summarized in the following information.

Mental Retardation

Down syndrome is the leading genetic cause of mental retardation, and there is a range of cognitive deficiency. A majority of IQ scores are reported to be between 30 and 60 (Batshaw, 1997; Jung, 1989). General cognitive abilities appear to be better than general language skills in Down syndrome. Multiple developmental brain abnormalities are reported, including delayed myelination, fewer neurons, and neuro-chemical abnormalities in the neurotransmitter systems of both the central and peripheral nervous systems that cause impairment in synaptic transmission. Seizures are common in infancy and adulthood, and there is a predisposition toward Alzheimer disease as individuals with Down syndrome grow older.

Health Issues

Specific medical problems are associated with Down syndrome. Cardiac malformations and congenital heart disease are reported to occur in 40 percent of the population (Jung, 1989). Endocrine abnormalities occur, including hypothyroidism. This hypothyroidism can cause weight issues in children due to the slowing of the metabolism. Gastrointestinal mal-formations can result in newborn poor feeding, vomiting, and aspiration. Orthopedic problems, possibly related to ligament abnormalities, can cause partial dislocation of the upper spine. Short fingers with a mild curving of the fifth finger and altered palmar creases (transverse) are seen.

Disorders of the blood and a higher risk of developing leukemia are noted, as are skin disorders such as eczema. Obstructive sleep apnea is common due to the differences in the head and neck structures. Neo-plasias, benign or malignant growths, are seen in Down syndrome and can interfere with normal functioning of many of the body's systems. Their effect will depend on where they are growing and how quickly.

Physical characteristics

Persons with Down syndrome exhibit physical features that are recognizable across gender and race. Short stature is evidenced, with the average height in the adult male being five foot and the average female four and one-half feet. Generalized hypotonia is common and may result in hyperextendable joints. Vision difficulties, including refractive errors, tear duct obstruction, strabismus, nystagmus, cataracts, droopy eyelids, and inflammation of the eyelid, have all been noted. Early identification of vision disorders is essential and recommended as early as six months of age.

Dental issues have been identified in this population, with a wide range of problems. An early onset of periodontal disease with a history of rapid progression is seen, and gingivitis (gum inflammation) and loss of alveolar bone can result. Missing teeth, fused teeth, microdontia, and late tooth eruption of both the primary and permanent teeth are all exhibited. There are fewer cavities in the population with Down syndrome than in the general population. Malocclusions are very common, including open bite and posterior cross bite, and these dental abnormalities significantly affect speech production.

Facial Features

Children with Down syndrome have specific facial features that aid in early identification. Brachycephaly (shortness of the anterior to posterior diameter of the skull) is exhibited, with a flat facial profile. A small nose and chin are seen, with a tendency toward protrusion of the tongue. Epincanthal folds and upslanting palpebral fissures (opening between the upper and lower eyelid) are distinctive in Down syndrome, as are Brushfield

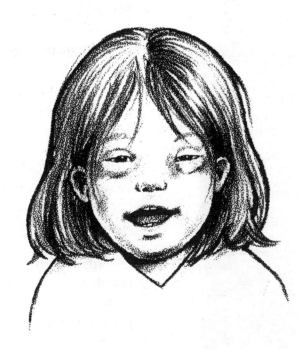

spots, a speckling of the iris. Excess skin on the back of the neck and small ears are also seen with possible anomalies such as an absent earlobe or an overfolding of the upper auricle edge.

Speech-Language Issues

- Oral Motor/Articulation

- Hearing

- Dysfluency

- Voice

- Language

Speech-Language Issues . . . .

There are significant speech-language delays and disorders noted with Down syndrome. The oral-motor structure, hypotonia, and degree of mental retardation all play a part in the degree to which speech and language develop in each child. Hearing abilities are also a major factor to consider in this population.

Oral Motor/Articulation

A major area of concern within speech-language issues for people with Down syndrome is the entire oral-motor and articulatory arena. The oral structure in Down syndrome is characteristic, with an open bite, a posterior cross bite, and other malocclusions observed. A large, protruding tongue is noted, even by the casual observer, and may seem even more enlarged due to the accompanying small oral opening and small chin. The restriction of tongue movement within a smaller oral cavity with a narrow palate affects speech articulation. Multiple neuromuscular anomalies can contribute to tongue control difficulties and problems with positioning for phoneme production. Generalized hypotonia can also be an influencing factor.

The onset and development of meaningful speech in children with Down syndrome is delayed and, although these children may be identified as having phonological processing disorders or traditional articulatory disorders, a major presenting characteristic is overall speech unintelligibility. This delayed onset of speech and labored articulation, in addition to inconsistent error patterns, possibly due to structural differences and hypotonia, can result in very poor speech intelligibility. Couple this with voice quality disorders and dysfluencies, and you have a client who is most difficult to understand, even to the familiar interactional partner. Kumin (1994) also noted the existence of dysarthria and verbal apraxia in the population.

Hearing

A majority of children with Down syndrome experience difficulties in the hearing area, up to 75 per cent of the population. Small auricles with an overfolding of the helix of the pinna may be noted by the casual observer. Conductive hearing losses are most common, with impacted cerumen and middle-ear infections accounting for the majority of difficulties. These conductive losses can be unilateral or bilateral. Narrowing of the naso-pharynx, malformation of the Eustachian tube, and susceptibility to upper respiratory infections can contribute to middle-ear infection. Chronic middle-ear infections can lead to destruction of the ossicles, and some children are born with ossicular malformations, which are not efficient in transmitting sound waves to the inner ear. Tympanometric audiometry techniques are efficient at identifying the status of the middle ear and are recommended at frequent intervals due to the prevalence of middle-ear infection in the population.

Sensorineural losses are also noted in children with Down syndrome, and they can be unilateral or bilateral. Early identification of these losses is essential, beginning with auditory brainstem response testing that is recommended by six months of age.

Dysfluency

Fluency difficulties are seen in Down syndrome, but the jury is still out as to whether these are speech based or language based. In addition to the dysfluencies, occasional bursts of rapid speech have also been exhibited. The dysfluencies can be an additional factor contributing to the high levels of unintelligibility seen in this population.

Voice

Vocal quality disturbances are exhibited by children with Down syndrome, and a breathy, husky voice with a low pitch may be heard. Hypernasality with nasal air emissions may also be heard. The generalized hypotonia may account for some of these voice problems,

Intervention Issues

- Early Intervention

- Language Stimulation

- Oral-Motor Exercises

- Voice, Articulation, and Fluency Therapy

- Pragmatics

- Hearing

- Team Approach

particularly hypernasality and intraoral pressure difficulties if the velopharyngeal mechanism is involved. Structural differences may also play a part, as a high, arched, narrow palate can be exhibited, and the possibility of cleft palate and submucous clefting exists.

Structural differences in the head and neck region can also result in hyponasality. Lymphoid tissues obstruction and shortened oral pharyngeal structures are at fault and can also interfere with airway breathing. Obstructive sleep apnea has been reported for the same causative factors.

Language

Significant language delays with severe impairments are not uncommon in Down syndrome. Expressive language or language production is reported to be more involved than receptive language or comprehension skills, though both are affected. General cognitive abilities appear to be better than language abilities in the population.

Disorders in language comprehension are further complicated by poor verbal short-term memory skills, which affect the ability to comprehend instructions. The development of the first true words may be delayed as late as 24 months, with continued delays in the onset of multi-word utterances and syntactic development. Syntax development seems to be more seriously impaired than vocabulary and lexical development. People with Down syndrome are often observed to have an affectionate nature. Pragmatically, this can cause difficulties in interacting with others appropriately. Even nonverbal pragmatic behaviors such as the use of proximity, or the spaces between people, can be viewed as being inappropriate.

Intervention Issues . . . .

Federal law mandates early intervention services for children with Down syndrome. The following information summarizes major intervention issues for this population.

Early Intervention

- Children with Down syndrome are one of the populations eligible for early intervention services from birth. The high association of developmental delays in the population allows for early referral and treatment, and the efficacy of early intervention is good.

- Develop attachment and interaction with caregivers as an initial goal. Joint attention, joint action, imitation by caregiver of infant vocalizations and gestures, and mapping intent are all early skills that the speech-language pathologist can model for the caregiver.

- Addressing the above goals within the normal daily routine of the baby in the home is recommended. Caregivers should not feel as though they must break out time every day for "speech-language therapy." Rather, the daily routines of bathing, feeding, playing, diapering, etc., should be embedded with communication interactions.

- Play early socio-communicative games with the baby to establish eye contact and turn taking. Peek-a-Boo, So Big, "The Wheels on the Bus," and other early games, songs, and finger plays will stimulate baby and caregiver interactions.

Language Stimulation

- Indirect language stimulation techniques are one sort of language stimulation to provide for a young child. Parallel talk, self talk, and expansions (previews of the next developmental steps) are all techniques to which the child is not expected to respond. Rather, little bits of language are given to him in small doses throughout the day to help him learn that all things have a name, and to assist with cognitively "figuring it all out." Modeling is another technique to present a speech-language model to a developing child.

- Reading to young children allows for language stimulation. Preliteracy activities allow the young child to experience print and make associations between print and spoken words. Books with repeating choruses are often quite enjoyable as the child may be able to "chime in" during the frequent verbalization of a repeated phrase, such as *too hot, too cold,* and *just right* from *The Three Bears.*

Oral-Motor Exercises

- Imitation skills, including gross-motor, fine-motor, and oral-motor skills, are important for any young child to accomplish, as imitation is an essential learning tool. Tongue, lip, and mandible movements can all be seen and, therefore, are appropriate targets for imitation.

- Try blowing exercises to develop oral musculature and oral air control. Fun blowing activities such as blowing cotton balls across a space, with or without a straw, can be attempted, as well as whistles, pin-wheels, and bubbles.

- An occupational therapist might also be helpful in targeting oral-motor movements.

Voice, Articulation, and Fluency Therapy

- Voice therapy is often begun only following the examination of the patient by an otorhinolaryngologist (ear, nose, and throat doctor). The velopharyngeal mechanism and vocal cords must be observed and found to be treatable, or voice therapy may be indicated following surgical removal of tonsils and adenoids.

- Articulation therapy can take the form of traditional speech sound training, or phonological process therapy, where linguistic rule use is taught. Either treatment should address the overall speech unin-telligibility found in the population.

- Tongue reduction surgeries have been attempted to improve speech intelligibility in Down syndrome, but they have not been found to significantly improve articulation (Miller & Leddy, 1998).

- A determination of the dysfluency factors in each individual needs to occur, with appropriate therapeutics to follow. Is the dysfluency speech-based? Is the dysfluency language-based? If speech-based, will traditional fluency methods be appropriate? If language-based, would a program addressing dysnomia be more appropriate?

Pragmatics

- Pragmatic skill training is one of the lifespan issues for persons with Down syndrome. As expectations in social language use change with age, so should pragmatic skill training reflect chronological age appropriateness.

- Nonverbal skills, such as proxemics, gestures, facial expression, eye contact, body language, appropriate touch, etc., can be taught. Visual and physical cues can be useful here. For example, "We stand at least an arm's length away from another person when we are having a conversation." Use your arm as a physical cue.

- Verbal pragmatic skills can also be taught. Turn-taking, topic choices and maintenance, register, and appropriate language for various settings and interactions can be role-played, videotaped, critiqued, and utilized extensively.

Hearing

- Hearing loss can have such a detrimental effect on language and education achievement that early identification is critical. Because of the high correlation between children with Down syndrome and hearing loss, consistent monitoring and retest schedules are important to coordinate between family and hearing professionals such as audiologists. Monitoring every six months up to eight years is recommended.

- Frequent tympanograms can assist in the determination of the status of the middle ear.

- Family and team education about hearing loss and its effects is essential.

Team Approach

- Medical team members can include cardiologists, otolaryngologists, neurologists, pediatric nurse practitioners, and any other professionals needed to adequately address the many medical issues found in conjunction with Down syndrome.

- A physical therapist should address issues concerning gross motor, including the generalized hypotonia and hyperextendable joints associated with this syndrome.

- An audiologist is a key team member, due to the high correlation of hearing loss, both of the conductive and sensorineural types.

- Family members are important team members, particularly with the large number of children who are identified and begin services as infants.

- Occupational therapy is needed for fine-motor and sensory issues. Oral-motor and feeding issues should also be addressed by this professional.

- Psychologists are beneficial, due to the late onset psychosis and early onset of Alzheimer's disease seen in this population.

Summary Comments . . . .

Down syndrome is a definitive group of characteristics and symptoms known to have a common cause in the trisomy of chromosome 21. Down syndrome occurs across gender and race and is the leading genetic cause of mental retardation. Many medical conditions are associated with Down syndrome, as are sensory issues, including hearing loss. Speech-language development is delayed in the population, and this developmental domain is critical for young children. Early intervention services are made available for children with Down syndrome by federal mandate and are recommended to enhance development in all domains. A team approach including medical and educational professionals is beneficial to this population.

References

Batshaw, M. *Children with Disabilities, Fourth Edition.* Baltimore, MD: Brookes Publishing Co., 1997.

Jung, J. *Genetic Syndromes in Communication Disorders.* Austin, TX: Pro-Ed, 1989.

Kumin, L. *Communication Skills in Children with Down Syndrome: A Guide for Parents.* Rockville, MD: Woodbine House, 1994.

Mervis, C. B., and Bertrand, J. "Developmental Relations Between Cognition and Language: Evidence from Williams Syndrome." In L. B. Adamson and M. A. Romski (Eds.) (pp. 75-107). *Communication and Language Acquisition: Discoveries from Atypical Development.* Baltimore, MD: Brookes Publishing Co., 1997.

Miller, J. F., and Leddy, M. "Down Syndrome: The Impact of Speech Production on Language Development." In R. Paul (Ed.) (pp. 163-177). *Exploring the Speech-Language Connection.* Baltimore, MD: Brookes Publishing Co., 1998.

Paul, R. *Language Disorders from Infancy Through Adolescence: Assessment and Intervention.* St. Louis: Mosby-Year Book, Inc., 1995.

Shprintzen, R. J. *Genetics, Syndromes and Communication Disorders.* San Diego: Singular Publishing Group, Inc., 1997.

Fetal Alcohol Syndrome

Characteristics

- Prenatal and postnatal growth retardation
- Central nervous system dysfunction
- Craniofacial abnormalities

- due to mother's drinking during pregnancy

- low birth weight

- "failure to thrive"

- language and learning difficulties

- 1/1,000 to 1/2,400

Syndrome Definition . . . .

Fetal alcohol syndrome is comprised of a group of physical findings that result from maternal consumption of alcohol during pregnancy. Sparks (1993) calls the diagnosis of fetal alcohol syndrome a clinical judgment, as there are no lab tests available for definitive diagnosis. The timing and duration of the alcohol consumption during pregnancy vary from expectant mother to expectant mother, thus the effects of the alcohol vary from child to child. Also, because alcohol can affect any developmental process in the growing fetus, the variances of both physical and behavioral features can be staggering. Fetal alcohol syndrome has even been associated with binge drinking during pregnancy. Because alcohol is such a strong teratogen to the developing embryo and fetus, alcoholic drinks now carry a label warning pregnant women not to drink; the ethyl alcohol in these beverages has been found to cause birth defects.

The diagnosis of fetal alcohol syndrome (FAS) is most often based on three broad categories of criteria. These include prenatal and postnatal growth retardation, central nervous system abnormalities, and craniofacial abnormalities (Batshaw, 1997). In the following section, specific characteristics within each category will be discussed.

There are also children who display fetal alcohol effect (FAE) who do not meet the specific criteria for a diagnosis of fetal alcohol syndrome but are definitely affected by the teratogen in utero.

Diagnosis may be difficult in young children, especially since many women who drink during pregnancy are not forthcoming about this behavior during the diagnostic process. Careful probing in the case history may be the only way to discover maternal drinking behaviors. Often women who drank during pregnancy also used illegal substances, and the diagnosis of fetal alcohol syndrome is made even more difficult due to polydrug use. One last difficulty in diagnosis is that many children with fetal alcohol syndrome do not remain in their birth homes, but rather enter into foster care systems. This circumstance may make it even more difficult to obtain accurate case history information.

The incidence of fetal alcohol syndrome is difficult to determine based on many of the same reasons that diagnosis is so difficult. Batshaw (1997) reported the prevalence number worldwide at one or two per 1,000 births. Jung (1989) put the number at .04 percent of births, or one in 2,423 term pregnancies. Higher incidences of fetal alcohol syndrome have been noted in various populations of the United States and around the world.

Behavioral Characteristics Profile . . . .

There are many specific behaviors and characteristics associated with fetal alcohol syndrome and these can vary widely in severity. These characteristics will be presented and discussed along the guidelines of the three diagnostic criteria for fetal alcohol syndrome:

- Prenatal and Postnatal Growth Retardation

- Central Nervous System Dysfunction

- Craniofacial Abnormalities

Prenatal and Postnatal Growth Retardation

Batshaw (1997) reported that babies exposed to prenatal alcohol are typically born at term, but that 80 percent have low birth weight. Seventy percent of these babies have severe feeding problems and often are diagnosed as "failure to thrive." Jung (1989) noted that the eye, head, and facial regions show more problems than the general skeletal growth. Microcephaly and cervical vertebral defects are both exhibited, along with minor limb and joint abnormalities. Though the children continue to be thin and of small stature in childhood, by late adolescence, they may achieve normal height and weight.

Central Nervous System Dysfunction

The effect of alcohol on the developing central nervous system is widely varied. Some children function in a range of mental retardation or developmental delay while others seem to be within a low-average intellectual range with specific learning disabilities. A greater degree of aberrant deformity has been correlated with lower intelligence quotient scores (Jung, 1989). Batshaw (1997) noted that two-thirds of children with fetal alcohol syndrome (FAS) display significant behavior and emotional disturbances. Batshaw (1997) reported that with fetal alcohol effect (FAE), milder intellectual and behavior impairments are seen with no craniofacial anomalies.

As infants, children affected prenatally by alcohol are often irritable and difficult to calm, and they spend a great amount of time crying. They may also develop tremors during this time. In a relationship with a primary caregiver, these behaviors may put the bonding of mother and child at risk. Temper tantrums can develop early, and it is not unusual for these to be recurrent, lengthy, and exaggerated.

As the children age, many additional behaviors are developed. These behaviors can include oppositional and defiant behaviors, strong will, little impulse control, no sense of danger, mood lability, lying, and stealing. The inability to govern their own behavior puts them at risk for developing reciprocal friendships and to live independently as adults. Inappropriate responses to social cues and the inability to understand consequences occur, and these children may be exploited by others. Social withdrawal, bullying, and anxious behaviors have also been exhibited. Perceptual abilities may be deficient, with the child having great difficulty integrating sensory information. Seizures of various degrees may also be present.

Children with fetal alcohol syndrome typically crave physical contact; they are friendly and gregarious with a true enjoyment of other people. They may encounter difficulty with interactions, however, as their social language skills may not be consistent with their expressive verbal abilities.

A lack of ability to make transitions as well as a lack of responsiveness to rules and directions make educational planning difficult with this population. There can be multiple difficulties in academic performance based on the cognitive deficit caused by the central nervous system dysfunction. Some noted behaviors consistent with the diagnosis include attention problems, hyperactivity, poor memory, poor judgment, and poor problem solving. These children may appear fast moving and full of energy and may not stay long at any one activity.

Difficulties with abstract thought and reasoning develop and mathematics may be a particularly challenging subject. Language-learning disabilities are noted, including difficulty in reading and writing.

Craniofacial Abnormalities

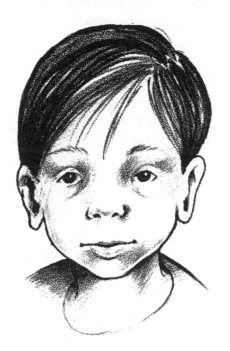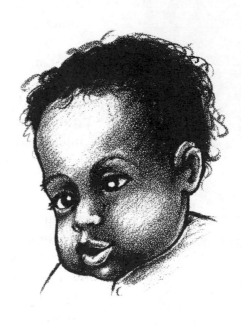

The craniofacial abnormalities within fetal alcohol syndrome can be quite distinct in the child whose mother drank alcohol heavily throughout her pregnancy. In other cases, the abnormalities may be less easily visible. Microcephaly is often noted, along with widely spaced eyes with narrow eyelids. The slit of the eye formed by the upper and lower lid, called the *palpebral fissure*, appears short in the child with fetal alcohol syndrome. A small, upturned nose with anteverted nares, a thin upper lip, and retrognathia (underdeveloped jaw) are also common. Clefting of the lip and/or palate have been exhibited, including the specific case of submucous cleft palate. The philtrum, or the groove in the midline of the lips, is flattened and appears to be large. A flat maxilla and shortening of the ramus of the mandible, along with midface hypoplasia (underdevelopment), are noted. Small teeth with faulty enamel and malocclusion are seen, and many of these craniofacial anomalies will affect speech-language development.

Ear malformation of both the pinna and the middle ear can be seen in fetal alcohol syndrome, and protuberant ears are not uncommon. Posterior

Speech-Language Issues

- Voice Disorders

- Articulation Disorders

- Hearing (frequent ear infections)

- Language Disorders

rotation of the auricle and poorly formed concha may be exhibited. There is a higher incidence of otitis media and sensorineural hearing loss in fetal alcohol syndrome, due to the neurotoxicity of alcohol to the developing brainstem and inner ear (Scott, 1998).

Other Physical Characteristics

There are other associated physical characteristics in fetal alcohol syndrome in addition to the craniofacial anomalies already described. A congenital heart anomaly, vetriculoseptal defect, has been observed in the population. Vision complications noted in childhood include strabismus, nystagmus, astigmatism, and myopia. Renal anomalies, hernias, and genito-urinary malformations have been exhibited, and these children have been known to be late to toilet train. In addition to primary microcephaly, Shprintzen (1997) reported a low anterior hairline related to the deficiency in the development of the frontal lobe.

Hypotonia and associate motor delays have been reported, with improvement in gross-motor skills with age; fine-motor problems may persevere. A distinctive palmar crease reported by Shprintzen (1997) appears as a single crease that runs across the palm and exits between the index and middle fingers.

Speech-Language Issues . . . .

A variety of speech-language disorders is associated with fetal alcohol syndrome, some of which also involve the hearing system. These can be based on the craniofacial anomalies, the central and peripheral nervous system dysfunction, or even the caregiving environment. The speech-language pathologist as part of an educational team can be very beneficial to appropriate programming for these children. The primary speech-language issues in working with children within this syndrome are explained on the following pages.

Voice Disorders

Resonance problems are common among children with fetal alcohol syndrome. Many of them have clefting or velopharyngeal insufficiency, and craniofacial anomalies have also been determined in this population. Hypernasality and nasal air emissions are most commonly heard. Treatment of the cleft, either surgical or prosthetic, may improve resonance. In the area of vocal quality, hoarseness may occur, and a high-pitched cry in infancy has been exhibited.

Articulation Disorders

Speech delays and articulation errors may be due to developmental patterns or may be secondary to structural change such as clefting and velopharyngeal insufficiency. Having poor feeding skills in very early life does not allow for the normal movement patterns necessary for adequate pre-speech motions to develop. The hypotonia noted previously may effect speech sound production. Dyspraxia has also been noted in these children. Since many of these children have craniofacial differences, such as dental malocclusions and micrognathia, articulation errors can be expected.

Hearing

Ear malformation of both the pinna and the middle ear has been noted in the previous section. A higher incidence of otitis media and sensorineural hearing loss in fetal alcohol syndrome exists and is thought to be due to the neurotoxicity of alcohol to the developing brainstem and inner ear and the craniofacial anomalies seen (Scott, 1998). The eustachian tubes and base angle of the skull in children with fetal alcohol syndrome have been found to differ from the norm, resulting in otitis media, and tympanostomy tubes may be inserted. Conductive hearing loss associated with otitis media may occur if untreated, and potential scarring of the eardrum may occur. Central auditory processing disorders have also been noted.

Language Disorders

Delayed and impaired language with global cognitive impairment in fetal alcohol syndrome has been reported by many sources (Shprintzen, 1997; Schoenbrodt et al., 1995; Sparks, 1993). Language consistent with cognitive levels should be expected, with difficulties in syntax, semantics, and

Intervention Issues

- Positive Caregiver Interaction

- Hearing Issues

- Voice and Articulation

- Functional Language

- Behavior Management

pragmatics. Impairments in language acquisition as well as language use are noted. Jung (1989) reported that the severity and subtypes of language involvement relate to central and peripheral nervous system damage.

Language is a system we use to communicate, and children need a strong child-caregiver environment for the development of very early language interaction skills. As has been noted, babies with fetal alcohol syndrome may be irritable and cry often, thus putting caregiver interaction at risk. The caregiver and the environment may also be nonconducive to caregiver-child interaction if the mother continues to drink alcohol and possibly abuse other drugs, or if the child enters a foster care system without a consistent primary caregiver.

Both receptive and expressive language abilities have been found to be deficient with fetal alcohol syndrome. The receptive disorders may present themselves as processing disorders, and the correlating attentional difficulties may compound these problems as do the memory deficits. The expressive disorders include delays in the age at which children start to produce words and begin word combinations; reported mean length of utterance (MLU) is below what would be expected for chronological age. Language-learning disabilities may manifest themselves in the early school years and can affect reading, writing, and mathematics.

Pragmatic language seems to hold particular challenges for children with fetal alcohol syndrome, with many skills being deficient. Difficulties around topic are frequent, including poor topic choice and topic perseveration. Questioning as a conversational strategy has been recognized, and echolalia can be present.

Intervention Issues . . . .

A speech-language pathologist is a primary team member in working with children exposed prenatally to alcohol. The speech-language disorders may vary in type and severity, and each child will present a unique profile. Early identification and intervention are critical to these developing children. Some common intervention issues arc summarized in the following information.

Positive Caregiver Interaction

- Techniques to increase attachment and interaction with the caregiver and the infant exposed prenatally to alcohol include some physical means associated with baby's states. In the child who cries whenever awake, it is difficult to have meaningful interaction, so techniques to calm the child may be called for. Swaddling in very close fitting wraps can help to calm the child, as can firm touch and low stimulation. Reading a child's signals for too much stimulation, such as breaking eye contact or distancing from an interactional partner, is another skill that a caregiver can be taught.

Hearing Issues

- Awareness and treatment of otitis media is essential in fetal alcohol syndrome. There is a higher incidence of otitis media, and this can result in a fluctuating conductive loss. Whether medical or surgical treatment is indicated, the status of the middle ear is of utmost importance.

- The anomalies of the outer ear do not interfere with hearing to the extent of middle ear anomalies.

- A higher incidence of sensorineural hearing loss is also common, and early identification once again with the teaming of an audiologist and otorhinolaryngologist is beneficial.

- Potential central auditory processing difficulties also call for teaming with a hearing professional.

Voice and Articulation Therapy

- Voice therapy to address resonance difficulties may be indicated following either surgical or prosthetic treatment of any cleft formations or velopharyngeal incompetence.

- Vocal hygiene programs can be initiated to prevent vocal abuses and misuses.

- Those abuses and misuses that are currently identified need to be reduced.

- Traditional articulation therapy is recommended for those phoneme errors not associated with craniofacial anomalies. Articulation usually improves with age and treatment.

Functional Language Skills

- Begin early. Early intervention, early childhood special education, Head Start, and at-risk programs all allow speech-pathologists to intervene with the youngest children experiencing results of prenatal exposure to alcohol.

- Specific support in a language development classroom or a resource room may allow for more functional language treatment than would itinerant services. A classroom setting could allow for the multisensory instructional approach where all types of language are targeted, including verbal, written, gestural, and nonverbal communication. Language treatment will depend on the functioning level of the individual. Concrete situations allow for true functional language use and should be built into the daily routine for these children.

- Pragmatic skills will need to be taught. Integrate specific behaviors relevant to social appropriateness with language therapy and possibly the academic program. Appropriate skills around topic issues; use of questions; choice making; and register issues, such as speaking to people according to status, gender, age, etc., could all be useful objectives. For younger children, teaching the intent and function of language use can be objectives.

- Target reading, writing, and mathematics within the framework of the language-learning disability. Teaming with a resource teacher can help the speech-language pathologist learn more about school curricula and the language demands involved.

- Consider life-span planning in intervention. "Where will this child be when his public education is finished at age 18 or age 21?" is a question we must consider if planning for functional language use.

Behavior Management

- Behavior management techniques will surely be utilized in any speech-language situation with children with fetal alcohol syndrome. Attention, concentration, challenging behaviors, memory difficulties, and hyperactivity are all behaviors for which the speech-pathologist must be ready. Motivating the child may be particularly challenging; consider using positive reinforcement techniques.

- Minimize auditory and visual distractions in the therapy setting.

- Physical management of the environment may be needed, with furniture positioned in a certain manner within a therapy room to decrease behaviors such as out-of-seat and temper tantrums.

- Use structure and repetition with established routines, such as going to McDonald's®, to prepare the child for a positive, functional outcome.

Summary Comments . . . .

Fetal alcohol syndrome (FAS) is a resulting condition from maternal consumption of alcohol during pregnancy. The three areas of diagnostic criteria include prenatal and postnatal growth deficiency, central nervous system dysfunction, and craniofacial anomalies. Each child affected by alcohol toxicity presents an individual profile, as the timing and duration of the alcohol consumption on the developing embryo and fetus varies per individual. Fetal alcohol effect (FAE) may present if all three criteria for fetal alcohol syndrome are not exhibited.

Children with fetal alcohol syndrome may be at risk for communication disorders due to their physical characteristics, their environment, or a combination of both physical and environmental characteristics. Caregiving interaction patterns must be considered in the very youngest children.

School-aged children also face difficulties. Learning problems are frequent in this population, compounded with behavioral difficulties. Attentional abilities, deficient memory, lack of concentration, and hyperactivity may all pose a challenge for the child with fetal alcohol syndrome or fetal alcohol effect. The speech-language pathologist is an important member on the educational team for these children.

References

Batshaw, M. *Children with Disabilities, Fourth Edition.* Baltimore, MD: Brookes Publishing Co., 1997.

Jung, J. *Genetic Syndromes in Communication Disorders.* Austin, TX: Pro-Ed, 1989.

Paul, R. *Language Disorders from Infancy Through Adolescence: Assessment and Intervention.* St. Louis, MO: Mosby-Year Book, Inc., 1995.

Shprintzen, R. J. *Genetics, Syndromes and Communication Disorders.* San Diego, CA: Singular Publishing Group, Inc., 1997.

Schoenbrodt, L., and Smith, R. A. (1995). *Communication Disorders and Interventions in Low Incidence Pediatric Populations.* San Diego, CA: Singular Publishing Group, Inc., 1995.

Scott, A. "Otitis Media and FAS." *Advance for Speech-Language Pathologists and Audiologists*, p. 5, August 17, 1998.

Soby, J. M. *Prenatal Exposure to Drugs/Alcohol: Characteristics and Educational Implications of Fetal Alcohol Syndrome and Cocaine/Polydrug Effects.* Springfield, IL: Charles C. Thomas Publisher, 1994.

Sparks, S. *Children of Prenatal Substance Abuse.* San Diego, CA: Singular Publishing Group, Inc., 1993.

Fetal Rubella Syndrome

Characteristics

- Deafness
- Blindness
- Central nervous system disorders
- Other physical characteristics

- due to German measles

- severity based on timing during pregancy; most severe impact during first trimester

- mental deficiencies

Syndrome Definition . . . .

Fetal rubella syndrome is the result of a virus also known as German measles, which causes an intrauterine infection. The virus is contracted by a pregnant woman. It crosses the placenta and affects the unborn child. Rubella was one of the first well-documented causes for birth defects as far back as 1942, and is a well-known viral teratogen. The virus is rarely noted in the adult, but has devastating effects on fetal development. The contraction of rubella during the first trimester of pregnancy will cause the most detrimental effects in the fetus, especially during the first six weeks.

Repeated rubella epidemics occurred up until 1969, when a vaccine was developed for rubella, and widespread inoculations began. Though the incidence of fetal rubella syndrome has decreased dramatically, it does still occur.

Behavioral Characteristics Profile . . . . .

The following information explains the major behavioral characteristics of children within the fetal rubella syndrome.

Deafness

Sensorineural hearing impairment occurs in fetal rubella syndrome. A bilateral or unilateral loss can occur, and can vary in severity. The child exposed to the virus in the first trimester of pregnancy will most likely have a severe to profound loss. This virus is known to infect the developing cochlea.

Blindness

A variety of eye anomalies is seen in fetal rubella syndrome, including bilateral cataracts, salt and pepper retinopathy (Jung, 1989), glaucoma, small eyes, and chorioretinitis.

Central Nervous System Dysfunction

Central nervous system dysfunction can vary in the child with fetal rubella, depending on the timing of the virus contraction that affects the developing brain and spinal cord. Mental deficiency is noted, as is difficulty with motor coordination and balance. Some of these children will be considered mentally retarded, while others may present a learning disability. Impulsivity, attention disorders, autistic behaviors, and poor school performance are all noted (Paul, 1995; Jung, 1989). Microcephaly has also been reported.

Other Physical Characteristics

Congenital heart disease and cardiac malformation can both be found in fetal rubella. Skeletal lesions as well as growth deficiency have also been reported, as well as the possibility for an enlarged liver (Shprintzen, 1997).

Speech-Language Issues . . . .

Hearing

As previously stated, sensorineural hearing loss of a unilateral or bilateral type are common with fetal rubella infection. The hearing loss or deafness will significantly impair the development of speech and language in the affected child. Jung (1989) reports that the sensorineural loss can be progressive, will be moderate to severe to profound, and will be relatively symmetrical bilaterally. Jung (1989) also reports that there are documented differences in the characteristics of the temporal bone in fetal rubella and a possible middle ear abnormality in the form of stapedial footplate fixation.

When speech is present in the child with fetal rubella syndrome, resonance and other voice qualities are reported to be within normal limits (Shprintzen, 1997). Speech may not develop, however, when the mental deficiency is severe to profound.

Language

Language development is impacted by two of the common characteristics in fetal rubella. One is the hearing loss or deafness, the other is the cognitive deficiency or central nervous system dysfunction. Language development is delayed and disordered in children with fetal rubella. Some children will remain nonverbal, and augmentative communication means may be recommended.

Intervention Issues . . . .

Consider the following issues in planning appropriate intervention for children with fetal rubella syndrome.

Team Approach

With the variance of severity seen in children with fetal rubella syndrome, it is difficult to give a prognosis for the entire group. Treat each child individually, with a personal profile of strengths and needs. A team approach with collaboration of medical and educational professionals and the family is beneficial. Early identification and early intervention are critical in light of the possible severity of the disabilities.

Monitor Hearing

- Fetal rubella syndrome has been associated with a hearing loss that can be of a progressive nature. Continued monitoring of the hearing mechanism, therefore, is essential. If a child has amplification, this assistive technology must be carefully monitored.

Primary Prevention

- Immunization of all children and immunization before pregnancy would be ideal. Avoidance of pregnancy for three months following the immunization is also recommended.

Augmentative and Alternative Communication

- Because many of these children will not develop verbal speech, augmentative communication means may be warranted. Complete a careful assessment of hearing, vision, cognition, and motor skills, due to the involvement of many systems in fetal rubella. Again, a team approach is beneficial.

- If a child has a dual sensory disability (deaf-blind), consider a tactile augmentative communication mode. A board with actual objects or symbols raised from a flat surface might suffice.

- Consider multimodal communication, using all systems available. A child may have some natural gestures, a few vocalizations, a distal point, or any other variety of communicative means. All should be honored.

Summary Comments . . . .

Fetal rubella embryopathy is caused by a virus which is contracted by a pregnant woman and affects her unborn child. The timing of the intrauterine infection will determine the severity of the deleterious effects. Deafness, blindness, central nervous system disorders, and medical issues have all been associated with fetal rubella syndrome.

References

Jung, J. *Genetic Syndromes in Communication Disorders*. Austin, TX: Pro-Ed, 1989.

Paul, R. *Language Disorders from Infancy Through Adolescence: Assessment and Intervention*. St. Louis, MO: Mosby-Year Book, Inc., 1995.

Shprintzen, R. J. *Genetics, Syndromes and Communication Disorders*. San Diego, CA: Singular Publishing Group, Inc., 1997.

Fragile X Syndrome

Characteristics

- Developmental delays/Severe cognitive impairment
- Distinctive facial/physical characteristics
- Hypotonicity and joint dysfunction
- Vision difficulties
- Associated behaviors (hyperactivity, anxiety, etc.)

- hereditary, genetic disorder

- "X-linked mental retardation"

- cognitive, behavior, and communicative disorders

- 1/1,000 male, 1/2,000 female live births

- milder characteristics among females

Syndrome Definition . . . .

Fragile X is a hereditary disorder that has also been referred to as *X-linked mental retardation* (Shprintzen, 1997). It is an X-linked genetic disorder in which the mother is usually the contributing parent, and the syndrome can be identified in successive generations (Schoenbrodt et al., 1995). A fragile site on the long arm of the X chromosome is the cause of the syndrome, with the abnormality causing the tip of the long arm to become narrowed (Jung, 1989; Batshaw, 1997). Fragile X can be identified with a DNA blood test for Fragile X. As recently as 1991, an underlying gene defect, an abnormality in the SMRI (fragile X mental retardation) gene, was found in all individuals with Fragile X (Batshaw, 1997).

Fragile X syndrome is second only to Down syndrome as a genetic cause of mental retardation and represents one-third of all X-linked causes of mental retardation (Jung, 1989; Paul, 1995; Batshaw, 1997). Males are primarily affected by Fragile X, though females with the syndrome have also been identified. The female population is less severely affected by the syndrome than the male population. Scharfenaker (1990) reported Fragile X incidence as one in 1,000 males born and one in 2,000 females born.

Behavioral Characteristics Profile . . . .

The behavioral characteristics found in the Fragile X profile are summarized below. These characteristics differ in the male and female populations.

Facial Features

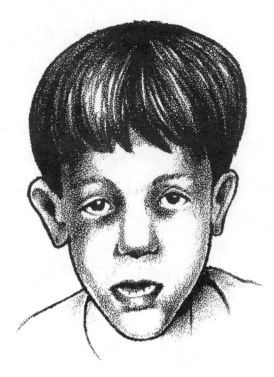

The distinctive facial features of Fragile X syndrome include an elongated, narrow face; a prominent jaw; long ears with abnormal auricles; macrocephaly; a prominent forehead; ptosis (drooping eyelids); and epicanthal folds. A high, arched palate and flattened nasal bridge have also been noted, and with that high-arched palate, an increased risk for cleft palate. These facial features are less exhibited in females with Fragile X.

Physical Features

The many physical features associated with Fragile X are, once again, often more pronounced in the male population. Hypotonicity and joint laxity have been noted, which can cause hyperextendible finger joints and other joints and can also cause poor coordination. A higher incidence of hernia and dislocated joints is reported, as well as mitral valve prolapse. Small hands and feet, flat feet, a mildly short stature, and macroorchidism (large genitals) are common. Vision difficulties, such as strabismus, farsightedness, and nystagmus, may also occur.

Mental Retardation

Most males with Fragile X syndrome exhibit a range of mild to severe mental retardation. This cognitive impairment can also affect females, but more in the area of mild retardation or learning disabilities. Girls may even present the facial and physical features of Fragile X syndrome, but may test within the normal range for cognitive functioning. Delayed motor and speech-language development is also noted. Each child presents an individual profile and may function better in certain developmental domains than evaluation would indicate.

Associated Behaviors

Hyperactivity, impulsivity, a short attention span, and discipline problems are all within the profile of a child with Fragile X syndrome. Self-stimulatory behaviors, tactile defensiveness, self-injurious behaviors, and tantrums have also been noted. A sensory-integration dysfunction is suspected in these children. This dysfunction may account for some of the associated behaviors, including the noted high anxiety. A late-onset psychosis has also been reported. Approximately 15% of children with Fragile X are also diagnosed as autistic or as having a pervasive developmental disorder, and most of these children are males. Although poor eye contact, withdrawal, and body orientation away from others have been observed, Fragile X children have also been described as *sweet, loving, shy, friendly,* and *eager to please.*

Speech-Language Issues . . . .

The speech-language pathologist needs to be aware of Fragile X syndrome and the variety of its speech-language characteristics. Communication skills may be related to the level of mental retardation being experienced by the individual child. Girls with Fragile X syndrome may be mildly impaired or may not present any specific communication deficits. These speech-language issues are summarized below.

Hypotonicity and Sensitivity

The hypotonicity noted in the children with Fragile X can exhibit itself in the oral-motor region. Initial feeding and pre-speech difficulties can be noted early on as these children are slow to feed or are poor feeders. Sensory issues, such as hypersensitivity or tactile defensiveness in the oral area, can also affect feeding and pre-speech movements. Hyposensitivity may also occur, resulting in drooling, mouthing, biting, or pica behaviors. Articulation development may be delayed due to the motor involvement.

Articulation

Articulation difficulties are noted in the population and may be associated with the level of mental retardation presented by the individual. Delayed articulation development is common, and oral-motor difficulties may be a partial cause. Shorter utterances are generally more understandable; as the child lengthens his utterances, he becomes more unintelligible. Dyspraxia has also been noted in this population.

Dysfluency

Children with Fragile X syndrome are noted to speak very rapidly, and this rate increases with their level of anxiety. Stuttering and cluttering have been reported, with common behaviors including frequent syllable repetitions and false starts. Intonation, rhythm, and stress patterns may also be disordered.

Voice

Though most children with Fragile X syndrome have a normal vocal quality, hoarse, breathy voices are not unheard of. Pitch disorders, lower than the norm in males and higher than the norm in females, can occur. The high palate formation associated with the syndrome should be carefully monitored to rule out the possibility of clefting.

Hearing

The hearing of children with Fragile X syndrome is generally within normal limits, but there is a higher incidence of otitis media than in the general population, and pressure-equalization tubes may be recommended. Also, due to the abnormal auricles and long ears presented by this population, extensive external examination of the hearing mechanism is recommended. Auditory-receptive memory and auditory-processing skills are generally deficient.

Language

Language comprehension and expression are related to the degree of cognitive function observed in the individual child. Receptive language and receptive vocabulary may be seen as strengths in children with Fragile X, though these will be affected by attention and sensory issues. There is some thought that these children may process information in a Gestalt mode, taking in "chunks" of information on which to build their cognitive concepts. This processing would account for some of the echolalia and perservative language noted with Fragile X.

Expressive language has been noted to be delayed in onset and progressive development and might not develop at all. In the case of children who do not develop expressive language, an augmentative or alternative mode of communication may be investigated. Perseveration and echolalia have already been noted, and pronoun reversals can be related. Word-retrieval difficulties have been observed, and language sequencing, organization, and syntax are poor. Verbal imitation is a relative strength.

Pragmatic behaviors, the social use of language, can be very inappropriate in children with Fragile X. Poor eye contact and body orientation away from a person are nonverbal pragmatic skills that can interfere with interpersonal communication. The lack of the use of gestures puts the listener at a disadvantage, particularly if the speaker with Fragile X is highly unintelligible. Topic maintenance is not strong, though turn-taking in nonverbal modes can be a strength.

In girls with Fragile X, a few higher-level language skills have been found to need attention, including abstract thinking, tangential language, topic maintenance, and narrative skills.

Intervention Issues . . . .

Early identification of Fragile X syndrome and associated early intervention is highly recommended. A team approach in the educational realm benefits the child in all areas of development. The following section explains some major intervention issues and goals for the child with Fragile X syndrome.

Sensory Integration

- Determine the best input systems for information processing (auditory, visual, tactile, etc.).

- Consult with an occupational therapist.

- Provide needed supports to maximize instruction and minimize interfering sensory input. Reduce visual stimulation in treatment settings. Offer choices for vestibular stimulation, including rocking, spinning, swinging, etc.

Oral Motor/Feeding

- If you are unfamiliar with oral-motor techniques, such as jaw stabilization and breakdown or oral defensiveness, consult with a speech-language pathologist trained in these procedures or an occupational therapist.

- Use oral muscle-strengthening exercises to decrease drooling.

Increase Attention, Decrease Inappropriate Behaviors

- Use behavior-management techniques such as positive reinforcement with tangible and token reinforcers paired with social reinforcement to increase desired behaviors.

- Ignore inappropriate verbalizations and behaviors.

- Use environmental control to decrease the opportunity for overstimulation.

- Be aware of medications being prescribed for attention disorders.

- Structure learning sessions with highly motivating materials.

Increase Pragmatic Abilities

- Role-play functional situations in which the student can practice appropriate topic choice, turn-taking, topic maintenance, and greetings.

- Increase appropriate nonverbal message modes, including eye contact, gesture, facial expression, and body orientation.

- Build on echolalia for turn-taking practice.

- Decrease perseveration; attend to the verbalization once and ignore repeated verbalizations. Reinforce the choice of a new topic.

- Consider the child's friendly nature, interest in peers, and good verbal-imitative skills in inclusive settings for pragmatic targets.

- Task-analyze social skills.

Increase Language Skills

- Use cueing systems for word retrieval, including initial phonemc cues, gesture cues, and visualization activities.

- Capitalize on good imitative skills to increase mean length of utterance.

- Generalize all skills to functional settings.

Augmentative and Alternative Communication

- For those children who do not seem to be developing expressive language, and for those children so unintelligible as to require augmentative means, another communication mode may need to be examined. Consider signing, gestures, picture boards, and electronic communicators.

Team Approach

- A special educator or a classroom teacher should generalize remediation and keep goals functional for the child.

- An occupational therapist should determine sensory-integration needs, oral-motor movement patterns, and special feeding needs.

- Consult an audiologist for otitis media concerns.

- A physical therapist will be helpful in positioning for learning and for issues arising from joint laxity.

Summary Comments . . . .

Fragile X is a hereditary, genetic syndrome that results in cognitive impairment, communication disorders, and behavior disorders. Males are affected more severely by the condition, with females exhibiting milder characteristics. Each child presents a unique profile, so educating these children can be a unique challenge. Many will present behaviors resembling autism, some of which may be based on sensory-integration issues, so a team approach is highly recommended.

References

Batshaw, M. L. *Children with Disabilities, Fourth Edition.* Baltimore, MD: Brookes Publishing Co., 1997.

Jung, J. *Genetic Syndromes in Communication Disorders.* Austin, TX: Pro-Ed, 1989.

Paul, R. *Language Disorders from Infancy Through Adolescents.* St. Louis, MO: Mosby-Year Book, Inc., 1995.

Sharfenaker, S. K. "The Fragile X Syndrome." *ASHA*, Vol. 31, pp. 45-47, 1990.

Schoenbrodt, L. and Smith, R. A. *Communication Disorders and Interventions in Low Incidence Pediatric Populations.* San Diego, CA: Singular Publishing Group, Inc., 1995.

Shprintzen, R. J. *Genetics, Syndromes and Communication Disorders.* San Diego, CA: Singular Publishing Group, Inc., 1997.

Landau-Kleffner Syndrome

Characteristics

- Normal general development, including language, for the first three-to-seven years

- Significant loss of language—first receptive, then expressive

- Abnormal EEG, with or without seizures

- Normal or above-normal nonverbal intelligence

- Behavior and sleep disturbances

- Inattentive to auditory stimuli

- extremely rare

- no apparent family history

- more males than females

- dramatic loss of language skills

- may involve seizures

- "acquired epileptic aphasia"

- may appear deaf or hard-of-hearing

- behavioral concerns

Syndrome Definition . . . .

Landau-Kleffner syndrome was first described in 1957 by the two physicians for whom it is named, William Landau and Frank Kleffner. The syndrome, considered to be extremely rare, is also referred to as *acquired epileptic aphasia*. *Acquired* aphasia implies that speech-language development is normal for a sustained period of time, but then a dramatic loss of previously acquired communication skills is noted. This dramatic loss of communication skills is the primary aspect of Landau-Kleffner syndrome. The main secondary aspect is abnormal results on an electroencephalogram (EEG).

Development is normal for the first three to seven years, with an acute interruption and regression of communication skills. Most cases demonstrate a loss of language over approximately a six-month period, but some very sudden, rapid regressions are noted. These children cannot understand or produce language that they previously produced and responded to appropriately. They tend to lose receptive language first, followed by regression in expressive output. Apparent lack of awareness or response to auditory stimuli can also be present as part of the regression, raising questions about hearing ability.

The primary neurological feature is the development of abnormal EEG readings, often discernible only in sleep conditions. A normal EEG in isolation is not enough to rule out the disability; other tests can be considered to substantiate brain abnormalities associated with Landau-Kleffner syndrome, such as PET (positron emission tomography), MRI (magnetic resonance imaging), or SPECT (single photon emission computed tomography) scans. The abnormal EEG patterns can be evidenced with or without the presence of seizures. About one-third of the individuals with Landau-Kleffner syndrome never develop seizures; medication can control seizures for those who do.

While medication can effectively control seizures, it has little or no effect on speech comprehension and behavior problems, which are assumed to be a reaction to the frustration encountered by the sudden loss of communication abilities. While autistic-like behaviors can occur, it is important to distinguish Landau-Kleffner from autism and other pervasive developmental disorders. Landau-Kleffner syndrome is not within the autistic spectrum, although a misdiagnosis of pervasive developmental disorder (PDD) frequently occurs.

The regression associated with autism occurs within the first three years and is marked by significant social isolation and lack of awareness and interaction, in addition to communication impairments. Landau-Kleffner syndrome does not present an autistic regression—it is primarily a language regression rather than a social one. In addition, the loss of language can occur without cognitive, social, or other autistic-feature regression. In Landau-Kleffner, neurological assessment yields positive results for abnormal EEG readings and/or seizures accompanied by significant regression in language. Individuals with Landau-Kleffner may be affectionate and retain normal emotional responses to situational stimuli, as opposed to the non-emotional, isolated affect typical within autism. The bizarre and extreme obsessions associated with autism are also usually absent or much milder within Landau-Kleffner syndrome.

Incidence figures suggest a rare occurrence of Landau-Kleffner syndrome with fewer than 500 cases reported worldwide. Males are affected two-to-three times (50-65%) more often than females. No consistent family history patterns are apparent within Landau-Kleffner syndrome. Theories to explain the disorder include a suspected defect in the temporal lobe of the brain, caused by auto-immune disorders, abnormal metabolism, viral degenerative brain disease, and effects of the repetitive epileptic charges.

The behavioral profile of characteristics associated with Landau-Kleffner is explained in the following section. It is important to remember that a normal developmental period occurs for minimally three years, followed by a significant loss of acquired language abilities the child has consistently demonstrated.

Significant Loss of Language

The primary distinguishing characteristic of Landau-Kleffner syndrome is a significant loss of previously-demonstrated language capabilities, both in receptive and expressive aspects of communication. The loss of language occurs for no apparent reason. Reported cases cite sudden changes over the course of a few days to a more gradual language regression over the course of several months. Severity is individual, occurring on a continuum from problems in articulating clearly to an inability to produce or understand language. Usually the child demonstrates trouble understanding and responding appropriately to language input. This phase is followed by a gradual reduction and regression in expressive language from production of complete sentences to telegraphic speech.

Receptive deficits range from difficulty following simple verbal commands to a complete inability to understand any verbal stimuli, appearing to be deaf. Expressive deficits range from misarticulation of sounds with a decrease in syntactic sentence complexity to a deterioration of using only single words, jargon, or mutism. Since their nonverbal intelligence is generally normal, these children often develop gestural systems to compensate for their expressive deficits. Sign language and other augmentative communication options have been effective in several cases.

Seizure Disorder

The cardinal feature from a neurological standpoint in Landau-Kleffner syndrome is the presence of an abnormal electroencephalogram (EEG). The irregularities may not be perceived during an aroused state; it is critical to also conduct EEG testing under sleep conditions. The convulsions or periods of "blanking out" reported by parents and professionals have contributed to the alternate name *acquired epileptic aphasia*. Two-thirds of the individuals with Landau-Kleffner syndrome will develop seizures, which can be controlled effectively with medication.

Behavior Disturbances

Aggression and temper tantrums are reported to escalate with the loss of language abilities. Children have been noted to attack others with various objects. Many of the aggressive behavioral components are attributed to the extreme frustration and confusion the children experience in response to the onset of language regression.

Hyperactive motor movement and poor attention as compared to earlier developmental patterns can be fairly dramatic in conjunction with the onset of the language loss. A diagnosis of attention-deficit hyperactivity disorder (ADHD) can result, but this diagnosis is not accurate when the full behavioral profile of changes is considered.

Landau-Kleffner is not included in the autistic spectrum of disorders because the key features of autism are missing from this syndrome. Autistic-like characteristics noted in conjunction with Landau-Kleffner include withdrawal, lack of eye contact, resistance to change, perfectionistic and compulsive tendencies in daily routines, picky eating habits, licking and smelling items before using them, and echolalia or telegraphic expressive-speech patterns. While these characteristics may be present, the intense lack of social cognition and awareness of other people and the environment, typical in autism, is not evidenced within Landau-Kleffner syndrome.

Sleeping patterns may also change dramatically with Landau-Kleffner syndrome. Children may have difficulty falling asleep, waken several times during the night, or require little sleep.

Simultaneous with the language loss, children may stop responding to auditory stimuli or appear confused when verbal directions are presented. Parents and professionals often suspect that the onset of hearing problems or a progressive hearing loss accounts for the changes in the child's language behavior. Most research suggests the continued presence of normal hearing acuity as measured by immitance procedures and evoked potentials. Despite auditory assessment results, apparent nonresponsiveness to sounds persists, and the child's actual voluntary responses to auditory testing can be variable.

Speech-Language Issues . . . .

Landau-Kleffner syndrome is an acquired aphasia disorder in young children, with a concomitant epileptic component. While behavior and medical issues are important, the significant loss of language abilities in a child who has consistently demonstrated language competence during the developmental period must take precedence. A speech-language pathologist is a critical professional in achieving accurate diagnosis and intervention within the Landau-Kleffner syndrome. The issues of concern are not diverse, but they are significant. They are summarized below.

Speech-Language Issues

• Aphasia

• Receptive Language

• Expressive Language

• Educational Concerns

Aphasia

Aphasia is a loss of acquired language. Intellectual potential is not compromised, just the ability to symbolically understand and use language. Adults and children who experience aphasia do not lose the capacity to think and reason. This intact cognition can lead to a variety of negative behaviors as a result of the frustration and confusion.

Receptive Language

Language develops in a child first receptively, with the ability to understand verbalizations within the environment, and then expressively, with the ability to verbally respond. In Landau-Kleffner syndrome, a child experiences a significant loss or regression of language in that same order. The child is confused by verbalization heard in the environment and gradually loses the ability to expressively respond to that auditory stimuli.

Expressive Language

As a result of reduced language skills, children with Landau-Kleffner begin to lose precision in expressive language production. Verbal output is often simplified to a telegraphic nature, with only main content words generated. Vocal production may also lose precision, as noted by a monotone speech tone and increased nasal resonance. Integrity of articulation can also be compromised as a result of the language regression. Phonological simplification patterns of final consonant deletion and metathesis (interchanging phonemes as in *aminal*

Intervention Issues

• Receptive Language
  Comprehension and
  Processing

• Expressive Language
  Production

• Team Approach

for *animal*) occur with regularity among this population. Children with Landau-Kleffner syndrome tend to be very visually alert and responsive to the use of sign language and gestures. Consequently, alternative augmentative forms of communication can be very effective in compensating for the language disability, as well as helping the child regain lost language skills.

Educational Concerns

Hyperactivity and behavior problems further complicate the profile of Landau-Kleffner syndrome. Poor attention, withdrawal, aggression, etc., all contribute to compromising academic performance. Regular education often has to be modified to meet the needs of children with this syndrome, particularly when in the regression phase of losing language.

Intervention Issues . . . .

A speech-language pathologist is the key professional in intervention efforts for Landau-Kleffner syndrome. While medical issues and treatment need to be addressed and coordinated, the primary feature is the loss of language that was previously acquired. Intensive services should begin immediately to recoup language abilities that were suddenly lost. General techniques can follow methods used within aphasia therapy, but should be modified to interest and motivate young children. The following information summarizes the primary issues and goals the speech-language pathologist should address within the syndrome of Landau-Kleffner.

Receptive Language Comprehension and Processing

• Evaluate the understanding of language input continually in everyday situations. Introduce functional vocabulary items for the child.

- Multimodality teaching (visual, tactile, and verbal stimulation) will enhance learning and clarify meaning.

- Use gestures and signs to supplement verbal input to clarify and improve the child's opportunity to attach meaning and understand the information presented.

- Introduce compensatory cues to teach the child to compensate for word-retrieval deficits and to highlight accuracy as the goal in language.

- Alleviate time pressures to reduce frustration. Encourage the child to focus effort to understand the language presented.

- Simplify verbal language to decrease processing and memory demands, such as one-step directions rather than several steps combined.

- Address conceptual language processing in a hierarchy of increased complexity, beginning with simple nouns and progressing to more abstract language concepts.

- Coordinate classroom modifications to insure learning and comprehension while minimizing the child's frustration.

Expressive Language Production

- Explore and develop alternative augmentative communication forms, based on the child's cognitive level of performance and residual language capabilities.

- Explore sign language or a total communication approach within the educational setting to enhance the clarity of language input and to augment language output.

- Work to continue expressive language production, expanding verbal output following the regressive state. For example, if the child has regressed to single words, begin expanding to simple phrases, telegraphic speech, and simple sentences.

- Evaluate phonological production to determine whether simplification processes are occurring, such as final consonant deletion and metathesis.

- Monitor the speech production aspects of voice production and address any concerns as necessary. For example, you could target a monotone voice pattern by exploring vocal inflection through retelling children's stories with characters of varying pitches and intensity, such as *The Three Bears* or *Three Billy Goats Gruff*.

Team Approach

- An audiologist should conduct evaluations, including evoked potentials and acoustic immitance, to assess hearing acuity.

- A psychologist should document the child's nonverbal cognitive performance level for assistance in educational programming.

- Psychology or psychiatry may need to be involved in counseling services to help the child understand and cope with the changes due to communicative loss.

- Neurology specialists should conduct periodic EEGs to monitor the status of seizures and irregularities in brain patterns.

- A physician or neurologist should monitor the use of anticonvulsant drugs and/or corticosteroid medications or other medical treatments.

- A special education teacher or hearing specialist may want to consider using an FM system or auditory-controlled listening environment to maximize the auditory signal.

- An occupational therapist may be involved to evaluate and program for fine-motor deficits that impact handwriting and visual-spatial skills.

- A physical therapist may be involved to evaluate and program for gross-motor deficits, particularly in walking/gait.

Summary Comments . . . .

Landau-Kleffner syndrome is a disability synonymous with acquired epileptic aphasia. A young child experiences a normal period of language development (minimally three years) that is disrupted by a dramatic loss of previously demonstrated communication skills. This language regression can trigger a host of accompanying behavioral components, interpreted as a result of the language problems. In addition to the changes in language competence, neurological evidence supports abnormal EEG readings accompanied by seizures in the majority of cases.

Medical technology is making significant gains in treatment options for Landau-Kleffner syndrome. However, in order to be effective, early intervention is critical for recovery. Corticosteroid treatment needs to begin early and be administered at an adequate level for a sufficient length of time (Lerman et al., 1991). Speech-language therapy to immediately address language deficits is also imperative. Medical reports caution that if the aphasia has been present for over a year when corticosteroid treatment is initiated, it is quite possible that EEG reading will normalize without positively impacting the aphasia. It is theorized that longer abnormal seizure bombardment to brain centers involved in language decreases the prognosis for recovery of language skills.

This trend appears to also be true in regard to surgical intervention. One theory speculates that an epileptic lesion is created in the speech cortex, interfering with normal circuitry for speech during development. Surgical intervention, consequently, needs to occur before the age of eight years, or the possibility of reversing the effect is reduced or eliminated.

If speech-language pathology is coordinated with current medical technology, dramatic results can be achieved within the syndrome of Landau-Kleffner. With appropriate early treatment, numerous cases reported regaining language skills and functioning well within an educational setting. Statistics cite approximately 20% as having recovered, an additional small minority who improved but had mild-to-moderate residual effects, while the rest remained profoundly aphasic.

The obvious conclusion is that early speech-language therapy is critical to improving prognosis for individuals with Landau-Kleffner syndrome.

●　　　　●　　　　●　　　　●　　　　●　　　　●　　　　●

References

"An Interview with Dr. Isabelle Rapin." *The Advocate—Newsletter of the Autism Society of America, Inc.* July-August, 1995.

"New Surgical Treatment Offers Hope for Children with Rare Disorder Diagnosed as Autism." *Autism Research Review—Institute for Child Behavior Research,* Vol. 5, No. 1, 1993.

"Landau-Kleffner: An Effective Non-Surgical Treatment." *Autism Research Review—Institute for Child Behavior Research,* Vol. 5, No. 2, 1993.

Lerman, P., Lerman-Sagie, T., and Kivity, S. "Effect of Early Cortico-Steroid Therapy for Landau-Kleffner Syndrome." *Developmental Medicine and Child Neurology,* Vol. 33, pp. 257-266, 1991.

Tharpe, A., Johnson, G., and Glasscock, M. "Diagnostic and Management Considerations of Acquired Epileptic Aphasia or Landau-Kleffner Syndrome." *The American Journal of Otology,* Vol. 12, No. 3, 1991.

Prader-Willi Syndrome

Characteristics

- Hypotonia (decreased muscle tone)
- Cognitive deficiencies
- Obesity
- Behaviors related to educational planning
- Distinctive physical features
- Delayed language development
- Voice and articulation disorders

- spontaneous genetic defect

- central nervous system dysfunction

- 1/8,000 to 1/25,000 live births

- insatiable appetite

- short stature; small hands and feet

- high-pitched, nasal voice

Syndrome Definition . . . .

Prader-Willi syndrome is a rarely-occurring group of symptoms first identified in 1956 by Dr. Prader, Dr. Labhart, and Dr. Willi. This syndrome has been previously referred to as *Prader-Labhart-Willi syndrome*. The incidence numbers vary greatly for the syndrome, ranging from one in 8,000 to one in 25,000 live births (Kellerman, 1998; Batshaw, 1997; Akefeldt et al., 1997; Kleppe et al., 1990). This syndrome is lifelong, can be life-threatening, and affects all races and both sexes.

The cause of Prader-Willi in the majority of individuals (70%) is a spontaneous genetic defect in chromosome 15. This tiny chromosome abnormality is a small deletion, or other abnormality, of the long arm of chromosome 15 that can only be visible with high resolution karotype (chromosome analysis). This high resolution karotype stretches the chromosome so that the smaller deletions and rearrangements can be visualized (Shprintzen, 1997). In earlier times, the deletion was missed due to the inability of diagnostic procedures to view the abnormality. It is currently thought that the long arm of chromosome 15 from the father is involved. If a deletion on chromosome 15 from the mother occurs, Angelman syndrome will result (see Angelman Syndrome, pp. 9-17). Prader-Willi syndrome is the most common genetic cause of obesity that has been identified.

Behavioral Characteristics Profile . . . .

The primary characteristics and behaviors are summarized in the following information.

Hypotonia

Hypotonia, or decreased muscle tone, is observed early on in this population. In infancy the low muscle tone can lead to poor motor control, a weak cry, poor sucking and swallowing, and possible failure to thrive. Floppiness in the neck region is especially noted. Delayed motor development is continued through the early years, though failure to thrive is replaced by obesity and rapid weight gain after age two. These children are thought to get stronger with age, but their muscle tone remains lower than the norm throughout their lives.

Cognitive Deficiency

IQs for the population with Prader-Willi range all across the board, with reports spanning the spectrum from 40 to 105. The average IQ is most often reported to be about 70, which would be mild mental retardation, though many of these children appear to function lower than their tested IQ score. Some students are even reported to function more like students with a learning disability than like students with mental retardation. Most developmental milestones are noted to be delayed by one or two years, which could be referred to as a *global developmental delay*.

Obesity

Obesity is reported in 95% of persons with Prader-Willi syndrome and develops somewhere between ages two and five. This obesity is a result of the combination of an insatiable appetite (polyphagia) and a metabolism rate just 60% of what is deemed "normal." It is thought that this insatiable overeating results from a lack of the feeling of satiation, which can be attributed to an abnormality in the hypothalamus. Appetite and weight control are long-term problems and are a serious health threat. The compulsive eating behaviors can be accompanied by food searching, foraging, and stealing. Overeating is treated with diet, behavior management techniques, and drugs, including fluoxetine, naltresone, and popypeptide infusions. The stress of diet control with these children can be extreme and needs to be coordinated between home and the educational setting.

Behaviors

In early childhood, children with Prader-Willi syndrome exhibit behavior somewhat immature for their chronological age. Stubbornness, noncompliance, difficulty with transitions, and temper tantrums develop in these young children and increase with age. Impulsiveness and disinhibition are also seen. Skin picking and scratching are noted and may be due to increased pain tolerance and decreased sensory input. Obsessive-compulsive tendencies may also develop, including concerns with symmetry, ordering and arranging, and perseveration on the same verbal statements and questions.

Physical Features

In Prader-Willi syndrome, there is thought to be a central nervous system malfunction that impairs body control, as well as a dysfunction of the hypothalamus that affects physical growth, sexual development, appetite, temperature control, and emotional stability. Apparent physical features include the previously-mentioned obesity, possible strabismus, myopia, and scoliosis. Short stature is common, with adult heights averaging around five feet tall. Small hands and feet are noted with tapering of the fingers and toes. Hypogonadism, or underdevelopment of the gonads, occurs and can assist in the early identification of the syndrome, particularly in very young boys.

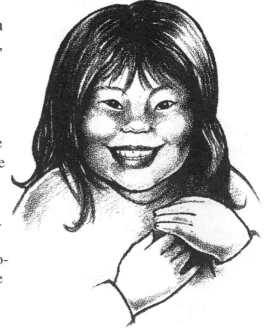

Facial features are distinct in Prader-Willi syndrome. A narrow palatal arch, micrognathia, an underdeveloped chin, and inadequate velopharyngeal closure may be seen. Almond-shaped, upslanted eyes and a narrow forehead are also exhibited.

Speech-Language Issues

- Voice Abnormalities

- Oral-Motor Dysfunction

- Poor Articulation

- Language Developmental Delay

Speech-Language Issues . . . .

Communication disorders are common in children with Prader-Willi syndrome, particularly in the areas of voice, speech, and language (Kleppe et al., 1990; Akefeldt et al., 1997). Although there are reports of poorly developed and low-set auricles of the ears, there is no higher incidence of hearing loss reported in this population. Hypotonia, which affects vocal muscles; cognitive deficiencies; excessive saliva; and the specific structural features associated with the syndrome combine as etiologies for the speech-language issues summarized below.

Voice Abnormalities

The early hypotonia of children with Prader-Willi can result in excessive hypernasality and a high-pitched voice. Nasal emissions and poor velopharyngeal closure are both exhibited and can cause phoneme distortions. The early hypernasality is reported to improve with age as the muscle tone increases and the structures are used more optimally.

Oral-Motor Dysfunction

Oral-motor ability has been found to be severely reduced in children with Prader-Willi syndrome. In infancy, low muscle tone affects feeding movements, which are also pre-speech movements. Once again, the hypotonia can affect the systems of speech production. Some evidence of flaccid dysarthria has been noted, and an above-average number of dysfluencies has been reported in the population.

Poor Articulation

Articulatory impairment is common in Prader-Willi syndrome. Both hypotonia and structural differences account for the difficulty with articulatory movement. The onset of speech can be delayed, and atypical articulatory skills can range from mild disorders to multiple articulation errors with reduced intelligibility. An inability to lift the tongue tip in forming the alveolar phonemes is a particular deficiency. Developmental apraxia of speech has been reported by some, but not all, researchers (Kleppe, 1990).

Language Developmental Delay

Since Prader-Willi is one of the syndromes that lead to mental retardation, language development is at risk (Paul, 1995). Comprehension and production of language are in accord with overall cognitive level, though receptive language may be more developed than expressive. There is a theory that a chromosome 15 deletion can lead to specific impairments in the language area, as seen in both Prader-Willi syndrome and Angelman syndrome. As noted with obsessive-compulsive tendencies, the child with Prader-Willi may have the compulsive behavior of asking or telling the same thing over and over, thus affecting the child's pragmatic language. Other specific language deficits include moderately reduced morphological and phonological abilities, including difficulties with comparative and superlative forms of adjectives, and a high percentage of content words found in language samples.

Intervention Issues . . . .

Intervention for the speech-language issues noted in Prader-Willi syndrome are unique to the particular behaviors noted. Early intervention efficacy is positive, and starting early with these children, their families, and other professionals in a team format seems to provide the most positive therapeutic results. A knowledge of the effect of the overall low muscle tone on the speech mechanism will assist the speech-language pathologist in making reasonable decisions regarding the early treatment of hypernasality and high pitch. Since each child with Prader-Willi syndrome presents an individualized profile for intervention, all skill areas need to be addressed. Ideas for goals and intervention planning are summarized in the following information.

- Oral Motor, Voice, and Articulation

- Behavior Management

- Receptive and Expressive Language

- Team Approach

Oral Motor, Voice, and Articulation

- Multiple articulation errors and reduced intelligibility may be remediated in part by oral-motor muscular strengthening. Positive outcomes for articulation can be achieved through strengthening the structure and knowing that the muscle tone increases with age in the population.

- Decisions regarding surgical treatment of hyper-nasality can also be put off while giving the oral-motor mechanism the opportunity to develop muscular strength to increase velopharyngeal sufficiency.

- Remediate accompanying flaccid dysarthria.

Behavior Management

- Use positive reinforcement to build new behaviors and increase desired behaviors. Social, tangible, and token reinforcers are recommended over food reinforcers.

- Use time out, ignoring, and/or stating of contingencies to manage noncompliance and temper tantrums.

Receptive and Expressive Language

- Increase both receptive and expressive vocabularies, emphasizing functional words.

- Improve syntactical and morphological proficiency. Strive for grammatical completeness in utterances.

- Use appropriate pragmatics in topic selection and decrease perseveration on compulsive repetitions.

Team Approach

- A physical therapist would address hypotonia in gross- and fine-motor movements. Assistance in increasing physical activity levels would also be helpful.

- Motor movement of the oral areas would be the focus of an occupational therapist. Feeding, swallowing, and sensory issues could also be addressed by this professional in collaboration with other team members.

- A nutritionist could assist a service delivery team in issues surrounding the obesity and metabolism issues common in Prader-Willi syndrome.

- A psychologist could address behaviors, including noncompliance, temper tantrums, food obsessions, impulsivity, and obsessive-compulsive tendencies. The education team would benefit from this input as well as the family members.

- Family members may be the most important members of the team in providing information concerning the day-to-day behaviors and routines of the child. They may also benefit from the services of other team members, particularly in light of behaviors.

Summary Comments . . . .

Prader-Willi is a relatively rare genetic syndrome that affects all races and both sexes. Obesity is one of the most commonly noted characteristics of Prader-Willi syndrome and remains a lifelong concern with this population. There is a cognitive deficit associated with the majority of persons with Prader-Willi, and language development will be affected by this cognitive deficiency. Hypotonia, or low muscle tone, is also highly associated with the syndrome and affects the speech production. Hypernasality, high-pitched voice, and articulatory disorders are all exhibited in the population.

Early identification of the syndrome is somewhat difficult, and reliance on physical features may be the first key to realization of a child having Prader-Willi. Hypogonadism is common in very young children and assists in early identification, particularly in males. Almond-shaped eyes, short stature, small feet and hands, and micrognathia (underdevelopment of the chin) may also occur.

Early intervention has been shown to be effective with these children in terms of behavior and communication. A team approach including professionals and family members results in "best practice."

References

Batshaw, M. *Children with Disabilities, Fourth Edition.* Baltimore, MD: Brookes Publishing Co., 1997.

Jung, J. *Genetic Syndromes in Communication Disorders.* Austin, TX: Pro-Ed, 1989.

Kleppe, S. A., Katayama, K. M., Shipley, K. G., and Foushee, D. R. "The Speech and Language Characteristics of Children with Prader-Willi Syndrome." *Journal of Speech and Hearing Disorders,* Vol. 55, pp. 300-308, 1990.

Kellerman, T. "What Is Prader-Willi Syndrome?," 1998. [Online] Available: http://www.azstarnet.com/~tjk/pws.htm

Paul, R. (1995). *Language Disorders from Infancy to Adolescents: Assessment and Intervention.* St. Louis, MO: Mosby-Year Book Inc.

"Prader-Willi Basic Facts and Medical Alert," 1998. [Online] Available: http://www.pwsausa.org/medalert.htm

Shprintzen, R. J. *Genetics, Syndromes and Communication Disorders.* San Diego, CA: Singular Publishing Group, Inc., 1997.

Rett's Syndrome

Characteristics

- Stereotypic hand movements
- Awkward, wide-stance gait; Ataxia
- Apraxia
- Mental retardation
- Seizures

- genetic mutation

- exclusive to females

- neurological regression

- unusual hand movements

- 1/10,000 to 1/15,000 female births

Syndrome Definition . . . .

Rett's syndrome was first described in 1966 by Dr. Andreas Rett (Gilbert, 1996). It is a genetic disability that appears to be caused by mutation of a gene on the X chromosome. At present, Rett's syndrome is exclusive to females; there are no reported male cases, suggesting an incompatibility with life in a male fetus. Incidence figures range from one in every 10,000 to 15,000 female births.

Early development is relatively normal for approximately the first nine to twelve months. Neurological regression begins at this point, and previously acquired skills are often lost. Predominant features associated with the syndrome are mental retardation, loss of voluntary hand movements, incessant hand-wringing movements at midline, apraxia, and seizures. These will be explained in more detail later in this chapter.

Rett's syndrome occurs within the classification category of Pervasive Developmental Disorders (PDD), which puts it within the spectrum of autistic disorders. While the initial diagnosis may be autism, as a child moves through the preschool years, differential diagnosis of Rett's syndrome becomes more obvious. There is good international agreement on diagnostic clinical criteria for diagnosis, as delineated in the *Diagnostic and Statistical Manual of Mental Disorders, Fourth Edition* (1994). *DSM-IV* diagnostic criteria are summarized below:

- Apparent normal prenatal and perinatal development; normal psychmotor development; normal head circumference

- Following at least five months of normal development, the following occurs:

  - deceleration in head circumference

  - loss of purposeful hand skills; onset of stereotypic hand movements

  - regression in social interaction

  - significant receptive and expressive language problems with an apraxic component

  - poor coordination of trunk and walking movements with ataxic components

Dr. Michael Powers further specifies the clinical features of onset in Rett's syndrome. The progressive, neurological regression can be divided into four identifiable stages, summarized in the chart on page 100.

Behavioral Characteristics Profile . . . .

Most of the behavioral characteristics associated with Rett's syndrome are listed on page 100. This section will highlight some of these components with a more expanded explanation. It is important to remember that a period of normal early development is interrupted by a flaccid plateau state, followed by a period of regression. Primary characteristics that constitute the behavioral profile of Rett's syndrome are explained in the following section.

Stereotypic Hand Movements

One of the most predominant features associated with Rett's Syndrome is the repetitive hand-wringing/washing gesture. An onset of self-stimulatory hand movements associated with autism gradually evolves

Onset of Rett's Syndrome

Stage One

- Developmental stagnation
- Deceleration of head and body growth
- Diminished interest in the environment

Stage Two (20-60 months)

- Increased deterioration
- Loss of previously-acquired skills in speech and cognition
- Loss of purposeful hand movements; hand wringing
- Apraxia
- Seizures
- Screaming
- Sleep problems
- Resembles autism at this stage

Stage Three (>60 months)

- Seizures
- Identified mental retardation
- Apraxia
- Ataxia
- Behavioral plateau
- Autistic features decrease; become more social

Stage Four

- Further deterioration in communication and cognition
- Decreased mobility
- Muscle wasting
- Dysfunctional breathing patterns (e.g., hyperventilation and breath holding)

M. Powers, 1998

into midline hand-wringing or hand-washing gestures in some females. Eventually the midline hand position is maintained, resulting in a loss of purposeful use of the fingers and hands. In other words, stereotypic, repetitive hand movements become less diverse and more consistently midline wringing when Rett's syndrome is present. Hand gestures typical of Rett's syndrome include clapping, squeezing, wringing, and washing.

Poor Coordination and Ataxia

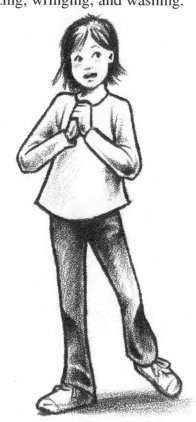

Both fine- and gross-motor movements become progressively worse during the stages of onset. Walking becomes stiff and awkward, moving towards a wide-based stance in gait with feet turned outward to maintain balance. Deterioration or atrophy of muscles is common as the child grows older, often resulting in scoliosis or deformities of the spine and limbs. Efficient, accurate voluntary-motor programming is significantly compromised, and ataxic aspects can result in limited mobility.

Apraxia

Oral-motor programming and coordination for producing speech regress significantly after the first year. A child may develop single-word production, but regression may result in a loss of these skills. Breathing irregularities, such as hyperventilation or breath holding, are also common within Rett's syndrome, further complicating the neurological aspects for speech production. Expressive language rarely exceeds a simple-phrase level of output, but early intensive intervention efforts are beginning to impact this area. While expressive speech is significantly impacted by motor aspects of the syndrome, receptive language is compromised by cognitive impairments typical of the syndrome.

Mental Retardation

Deterioration of cognitive abilities is a component of the degenerative regression during onset of the syndrome. Compromised cognitive skills impact the ability to acquire communication skills. Deficits in language

Speech-Language Issues

- Apraxia
  - Breath Control
  - Oral-Motor Strength
  - Sound Production

- Feeding/Chewing Issues

- Language
  - Receptive
  - Expressive

and cognitive ability have a dramatic impact on educational potential. Significant learning problems are typical within Rett's syndrome, and academic progress may be minimal, based on the degree of cognitive impairment.

Seizures

Seizures are reported in approximately 85% of the cases of Rett's syndrome. This epileptic component is evidenced in abnormalities on EEG readings. Medications can be prescribed in an attempt to control the seizures.

Speech-Language Issues

The speech-language pathologist needs to be concerned with several aspects of Rett's syndrome. They are summarized below.

Apraxia

Deficits in the ability to program movements of the oral-speech musculature can be profound within Rett's syndrome. The speech mechanism requires significant motor coordination of neurological systems involved with respiration, phonation, resonation, and articulation. In addition to poor motor programming, muscle weakness or atrophy can further compound the challenge of producing speech.

Disturbances in breathing patterns have a dramatic, disruptive effect on verbal output efforts. When the breathing patterns are irregular, the reciprocal coordination between inhalation and exhalation is disrupted. A controlled voluntary breath stream serves as the power source to initiate verbalization. When the first step is compromised, the process of producing speech cannot proceed. When significant breathing irregularities are part of the Rett's profile, producing more than single words or short phrases can be an unrealistic expectation.

If exhalation can be controlled and sustained, the next challenge is the oral-motor coordination required to shape sound into various phonemes. In addition to programming muscles to form consonant and vowel shapes in the oral cavity, muscles must have the strength and mobility to execute the neurological programming command. The muscle atrophy that often occurs during the regression phase of Rett's syndrome usually has a significantly adverse effect on the ability to articulate intelligible speech.

Feeding/Chewing Issues

Dysphagia, impairment in the ability to swallow, can be a concern in Rett's syndrome. If degenerative muscle regression continues, some children lose the ability to chew food, presenting feeding problems. Another aspect that can contribute to feeding problems is when purposeful use of fingers is lost to stereotypic midline posturing; the child is no longer able to feed herself, so someone else must assist. Oral-motor programming and muscle strength both contribute to difficulties in this area.

Language

Language comprehension is directly influenced by a child's cognitive level of functioning. A child with Rett's syndrome experiences a degree of mental retardation that impairs her level of receptive language development. Understanding will be better for functional, concrete vocabulary that impacts the child's everyday world. Abstract concepts, problem solving, reasoning, and complex language structures will not be attained by the majority of individuals with Rett's syndrome.

Expressive language is significantly impaired by apraxia and muscle weakness. It is critical to explore alternative augmentative methods of communication with individuals who evidence Rett's syndrome. Sign language is not a viable option due to the frequent midline, stereotypic hand movements. Written symbol systems are often too abstract for cognitive levels represented by individuals who have Rett's syndrome. However, a simple concrete communication system is essential to reduce frustration and establish interaction for basic needs and desires.

Intervention Issues

- Receptive Vocabulary

- Picture Communication Board

- Oral-Motor Exercises

- Swallowing Therapy

- Team Approach

Early intervention efforts should anticipate some of the residual components of Rett's syndrome. A speech-language pathologist might provide treatment during the regression or plateau phase of Rett's. Even though a loss of skills is possible, addressing anticipated deficit areas may serve to minimize long-term characteristics. Intensive early intervention efforts are beginning to modify the severity of some of the typical aspects within Rett's syndrome. The following section highlights the major issues and goal areas to address within Rett's syndrome.

Receptive Vocabulary

- To expand receptive vocabulary, bring functional objects within a child's everyday life to her attention and label them. Introduce vocabulary terms in categorical units emphasizing functional, everyday themes, such as clothing, foods, toys, etc.

- Keep language models simple so concrete terms for items are not lost in a complex sentence structure. Use telegraphic speech (only main-content words) to introduce language or communicative interaction.

- Multimodality presentation (visual, physical, and verbal) for teaching will improve the child's comprehension.

Picture Communication Board

- Explore alternative augmentative systems of communication that allow meaningful interaction.

- Make the pictures easily accessible to compensate for motor deficits.

- Pictures should be easily identifiable and objects that are high frequency in the child's everyday life.

Oral-Motor Exercises

- Respiratory control for breathing can be emphasized with blowing exercises utilizing party favors, kazoos, horns, etc.

- Emphasize oral muscle-strengthening exercises.

Swallowing Therapy

- Introduce exercises to strengthen the muscles involved in swallowing.

- Monitor chewing within functional eating situations to insure adequate muscle coordination.

Team Approach

- An occupational therapist may be able to address sensory issues in conjunction with stereotypic hand movements and other fine-motor impairments.

- Physical therapy may address gross-motor issues and ambulatory aspects.

- Respiratory therapy may assist with breathing aspects.

- Music therapy has been found to help breathing and motor speech patterning.

- Hydrotherapy, such as hot-tub therapy, can be very beneficial to address motor rigidity and sensory issues.

Summary Comments . . . .

Rett's syndrome is a relatively rare genetic syndrome that is exclusive to females. Following a normal pregnancy and early developmental period, development deteriorates and skills previously acquired are lost. Symptoms eventually plateau following an extensive period of regression.

Rett's syndrome is often misdiagnosed as autism between the ages of two to five years. However, as the regression continues beyond preschool years, behavioral characteristics tend to gravitate toward the primary features identified in this chapter (intense hand wringing and loss of purposeful hand movements, wide-stance gait, apraxia, ataxia, and seizures). Intervention efforts consistent with autism will not be detrimental, but differential diagnosis will allow remedial efforts to focus more constructively on features unique to Rett's. The disability is fairly involved in lifelong physical and cognitive aspects; an independent lifestyle is not considered a viable option at the present time, although early intensive intervention may eventually improve the prognosis.

●   ●   ●   ●   ●   ●   ●

References

American Psychiatric Association. *Diagnostic and Statistical Manual of Mental Disorders, Fourth Edition.* Washington, D.C.: American Psychiatric Association, 1994.

Gilbert, P. *The A-Z Reference Book of Syndromes and Inherited Disorders, Second Edition.* London, England: Chapman & Hall, 1996.

Powers, M. "Diagnosis of Autism and Related Pervasive Developmental Disorders." Eastern Illinois University Summer Institute on Autism, 1998.

Selective Mutism

Characteristics

- Social withdrawal or isolation
- Excessive shyness
- Oppositional
- Perfectionistic
- Speech-language deficits
- Body rigidity

- not genetic

- onset 3-5 years of age

- incidence <1/1,000 children

- responsive to early intervention

Disorder Definition . . . .

Selective mutism is not really classified as a syndrome disorder; however, it has multiple features which add up to the diagnosis and usually has an onset during the preschool years. Most speech-language pathologists have encountered several cases of selective mutism and were at a loss as to how to proceed. Early intervention is critical to resolving the disorder by elementary school age. For these reasons, selective mutism disorder was included as a chapter in this book. Note that selective mutism is not genetically determined and can be successfully resolved with focused appropriate intervention, unlike the other disorders in this book.

The disorder of selective mutism has been cited in the literature for over a century, but by different names. A German physician named Kussmaul recorded the first observations of the disorder in 1877. He described a disorder in which people would not speak in certain situations, despite the ability to speak, and named it "aphasia voluntaria" (cited in Dow et al., 1995). The disorder appeared in the literature from time to time without any specific label attached to it until 1934, when a Swiss child psychiatrist named Mortiz Tramer identified the characteristics as "elective mutism."

The disorder definition came from his belief that children were "electing" not to speak in certain situations and with selected people (cited in Harris, 1996).

The *Diagnostic and Statistical Manual of Mental Disorders, Fourth Edition* (1994) revised the disorder title to "selective mutism" to more accurately describe the disability. Rather than electing not to speak at all, individuals choose, or "select," situations in which or people with whom they will not talk. The diagnosis centers on a "consistent failure to speak in specific social situations. . . despite speaking in other situations" (*DSM-IV*, 1994). Selective mutism is included in the section on disorders diagnosed during infancy, childhood, or adolescence. Diagnostic criteria specified in the *DSM-IV* are summarized in the following chart.

Selective Mutism

- Consistent failure to speak in specific social situations despite speaking in others

- Interferes with educational or occupational achievements or social communication

- Failure to speak is not due to lack of knowledge with spoken language (e.g., foreign language)

- Failure to speak is not due to a specific communication disorder (e.g., stuttering)

Incidence figures suggest that selective mutism is relatively rare, with just less than one per 1,000 children affected (Wright et al., 1985). The gender ratio is slightly higher on the female side with about 1.9 females (58%) to one male (42%; Baltaxe, 1994). The age of onset is during the preschool years (three to five years of age) and usually occurs in the first educational setting outside of the home environment. The unfortunate statistic accompanying the age of onset is a referral age of six to seven years, meaning that opportunities for early intervention and resolution of the problem are often lost or compromised by a gap as long as three years. The disorder occurs across ethnic groups. Developmental language problems are an accompanying feature in the majority of cases (62-68%; Baltaxe, 1994). This is a significant variable for speech-language pathologists and will be expanded upon later in this chapter.

Researchers have been fascinated with the disorder of selective mutism for some time. Studies have explored a variety of family and individual variables that could lead to or cause a child to shut down verbal interaction in select situations. Maternal overprotectiveness, trauma, parental conflict, birth order, etc., are examples of variables postulated to explain the disability onset.

Subtypes of selective mutism have also been theorized, based on characteristics children have exhibited in various groups studied. A summary graph of differentiating mutism referenced in the literature is presented below and explained in the following section.

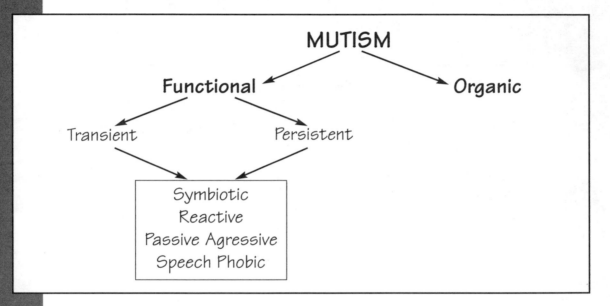

A primary initial differentiation is *functional* versus *organic* mutism. Organic mutism is attributed to an impaired central nervous system without psychological problems. For example, a child who has severe apraxia or cerebral palsy and cannot speak in any situation could be diagnosed as having an organic mutism. Selective mutism only includes individuals who demonstrate the ability to speak, yet choose when to use those capabilities.

A second differentiation mentioned in the literature is transient versus persistent mutism. *Transient mutism* implies the following:

- a recent onset of the condition (less than six months)

- child usually younger than five years old

- intermittent mutism

- mutism in one environment

Persistent mutism implies the following:

- mutism has existed longer than six months

- child usually older than five years

- consistent mutism

- mutism in more than one environment

The four subtypes of functional mutism usually mentioned are summarized below.

Functional Mutism

- **Symbiotic Mutism**
    - strong symbiotic relationship with caregiver, usually the mother
    - one parent dominates and controls relationships

- **Reactive Mutism**
    - associated with a variety of emotional reactions
    - results from single or multiple events that precipitate the mutism
    - considered more of a hysterical reaction phenomena

- **Passive-Aggressive Mutism**
    - child uses silence/mutism as a weapon or control mechanism
    - expresses hostility by defiant refusal to speak
    - often demonstrates antisocial behavior

- **Speech Phobic**
    - fear of hearing own voice
    - afraid of saying something inappropriately
    - obsessive need to control speech

Hayden, 1980, as cited in Baltaxe, 1994

The disorder of selective mutism was viewed almost exclusively within the realm of psychotic or psychological disturbances prior to *DSM-IV*. The disorder of "Elective Mutism" in the *DSM-III* was included within Axis II, which included psychiatric disorders. Professionals are beginning to acknowledge, as evidenced by the shift of inclusion in *DSM-IV* to the clinical disorders category, that selective mutism may not necessarily imply a significant psychological/emotional disturbance, but rather a developmental sensitivity to verbal interaction in select social situations. The early onset during preschool years also suggests a developmental problem that can be directly addressed in early intervention efforts. The goal is to intervene at the transient stage and remediate the problem during the child's developmental years.

Behavioral Characteristics Profile . . . .

Selective mutism has several characteristics associated with it. Despite the variety of subtypes and causes that have been theorized, the onset behavioral profile is fairly consistent in preschool children. Children usually demonstrate normal to high intelligence, evidenced by age-appropriate or advanced receptive language measures or nonverbal IQ results. Parents will describe a child who is fairly difficult to manage (e.g., manipulative and stubborn) in the home, while education professionals observe a child who appears isolated, shy, and reserved. Parents are often amazed to hear that their child is not speaking in a setting outside the home! The typical other scenario is a very shy, clinging child who refuses to separate from the mother in public situations. The primary characteristics associated with selective mutism are summarized in the following information.

Social Withdrawal or Isolation

Children exhibiting characteristics of selective mutism tend to observe from the periphery and withdraw from the demands of verbal social interaction. While somewhat isolated physically, these children demonstrate a keen awareness of the environment and are acutely vigilant in observing others' social interaction. They also show an astute awareness of levels in social demands, drawing a hard line at the level they are comfortable with and the level in which they will not interact. Some of these preschool children will nonverbally indicate their desires with aggressive, assertive pointing, but stoically refuse to interact verbally. Other children will participate nonverbally in activities, but will not eat in front of others, possibly not wanting to demonstrate any competency with the oral cavity. Even though socially withdrawn, children with this behavioral profile do not indicate the lack of awareness or cognizance of social demands that is often seen in autism. Children with selective mutism consciously choose their social isolation.

Excessive Shyness

Many children with selective mutism demonstrate extreme shyness in public situations outside of the home environment. They might maintain a very close proximity to their mothers, clinging to them and refusing to separate. Demands or social interaction directed specifically to one of these children may result in blushing or silent tears. Therapy often has to begin with a caregiver present in the room, with the caregiver's presence gradually faded as the child becomes more comfortable.

Oppositional

The other extreme of an excessively shy child with selective mutism is one who is extremely oppositional. Parents and teachers often describe these children as *stubborn, manipulative, strong willed,* and *controlling.* It is not unusual to observe a child refuse to comply or cooperate with directions given by a teacher or parent. The refusal is often accompanied by direct eye contact and a very stoic facial and physical posture. Interaction is often interpreted as passive-aggressive, with the child demonstrating intense awareness of the demand, but consciously resisting in a strong, silent style. It is almost impossible to trick these students into slipping up and verbalizing or responding to an interaction by accident!

Perfectionistic

A characteristic noted frequently in children with selective mutism is an intense desire to be in control and to make sure tasks are completed to their specifications. Nonverbal manipulation to accomplish their established routine is typical. These perfectionistic tendencies may feed the selective mutism to some degree, in that the normal intelligence and anxiety about doing or saying something wrong results in a stoic refusal to risk participation through verbal interaction.

Speech-Language Deficits

Research strongly suggests developmental speech-language deficits in the majority of children exhibiting selective mutism. The difficulties seem to be in expressive or output channels primarily, with normal receptive language and cognitive skills usually evidenced. The normal receptive comprehension results in an awareness of their deficits or differences. Rather than put a defective system on display, the children choose not to engage in verbal interaction. Typical deficits once the children become comfortable interacting are in articulation/phonology, pragmatics, and processing. Developmental apraxia has been noted in several children once the mutism has resolved.

Body Rigidity

Children with selective mutism can generalize the verbal interaction shutdown to a physical shutdown as well. They may withhold gross-motor interaction, as in playing on the playground, preferring to sit on

Speech-Language Issues

- Communication Hypersensitivity

- Evaluate Receptive Comprehension and Other Possible Speech-Language Deficits

- Expressive and Pragmatic Language

the sidelines and watch. These children may refuse to participate in physical education activities as well, refusing to run or comply with movement directions. Compliant movements are often very slow and plodding. Certain movements may be completely restricted. One child refused to eat or drink at school, waiting until he returned home to satisfy his needs!

Speech-Language Issues . . . .

Treatment options indicate that approaching selective mutism as primarily a communication problem has been successful. The role of the speech-language pathologist is critical in early diagnosis and intervention on this disorder. The disorder is not incredibly complex, but must be approached with a different perspective from the usual direct assault. The main issue is anxiety or hypersensitivity toward communication, accompanied by possible secondary speech-language deficits that are a source of embarrassment or frustration for the child. Receptive understanding and cognitive function are generally within the normal range. The speech-language issues are summarized in the following information.

Communication Hypersensitivity

It is important to acknowledge the child's sensitivity about communication without increasing anxiety. The child's perfectionistic tendencies convince her that it is better not to speak at all than to risk doing it poorly. Simple statements like "Sometimes it's kind of scary to talk to people you don't know very well" or " I'm not always sure what to say" communicate to the child that her feelings are natural. Modify your model to sometimes makes mistakes, whisper, and use simple sentences to remove some of the pressure on the child to imitate fully-developed, adult speech. It's also important to let the child know that, even though it is less scary and easier not to talk, it is necessary to talk; the child can gain more control of her world by using speech than by withholding it.

Become comfortable with silence. Many activities, such as drawing on the board or painting with water, don't require constant verbalization. At the same time, insert as many choices as possible for the child to control her world if she risks communicating. For example, if you are painting with water, have two pictures to chose from and offer her first choice. If she won't point, take the one you think she wants and give her the other one. This technique will increase her incentive to communicate the next time! Remember that most of these children are controlling, stubborn, and manipulative. It is important that they experience more frustration when choosing not to communicate than when they do interact.

Evaluate Receptive Comprehension and Other Possible Speech-Language Deficits

Evaluate the child's receptive comprehension formally to insure adequate language knowledge. Once a comfortable, consistent pointing response is obtained, administer a simple receptive vocabulary test to document comprehension level for general language development.

Through observation, note the child's social skills and comfort level for pragmatic interaction. Once single words are established, administer a phonological or traditional articulation test. The child will only be aware of naming objects or pictures while you acquire an inventory of phoneme development and competency. If the child's whispered words are unintelligible, incorporate oral-motor patterning imitation tasks to begin indirectly working on sound production.

Build Confidence in Expressive and Pragmatic Language Skills

Children with selective mutism often place unrealistic expectations on their own developing language systems because their goal is the adult level. The subtle social rules can be very confusing, so make them direct and less intimidating in a fun way. Play a game to do and say the wrong things and let the other person catch it. Read books and let the child drop a chip or clap her hands each time she hears *please* or *thank you.* Help the child practice and gain comfort with social interaction in a controlled, trusting environment.

Intervention Issues . . . .

Intervention Issues

- Establish a Hierarchy to Desensitize to Communicative Pressure

- Speech-Language Deficits

- Team Approach

Selective mutism is a disorder that tends to "fall between the cracks" in regard to who assumes professional responsibility for intervention. The condition is developmental and should be very temporary if remediation is appropriate. It is one of the few disabilities that can be completely erased if dealt with immediately at onset. If not addressed and allowed to continue through the school years, it can become severely debilitating with significant social and vocational ramifications.

Various therapy approaches have been attempted over the years to remediate selective mutism. Most that approached the disorder from a psychiatric viewpoint were minimally successful. Psychological counseling to discuss the anxiety puts a spotlight on an extremely sensitive area, causing children to retreat even further into their isolated worlds. Drug therapies have been tried with some success in older clients, but these seem to mask the real issue by medicating the individual to feel less anxiety rather than resolve the anxiety. Therapy that worked on building tolerance toward communicative pressure through positive reinforcement and pleasant play activities in a controlled hierarchy of increased verbal demand have been the most successful—and seem to make the most sense!

When approached from a perspective of anxiety toward communication, desensitization techniques logically follow. These intervention approaches are well documented in fluency cases, going back to the Van Riper era. Preschool children with whom this technique has been used have been successful in establishing comfortable verbal interaction in 100% of the cases in as few as six weeks of therapy. Often parents or teachers wonder how to get these children to stop talking once they start! As the child becomes older, the progression takes longer because the child has been allowed to function without needing to communicate verbally. The older the child, the longer therapy takes and the worse the prognosis for resolving the problem.

The speech-language pathologist should assume leadership in resolving selective mutism. The child needs to bond one-on-one with an adult who will "play games" and engage in motivating, nonthreatening activities. The child has to trust that person and form a bond. Within an isolated setting, that person begins a desensitization process. Once a child achieves a comfortable level of inter-action at one step in the hierarchy, then the expectation moves outside the therapy room while the adult begins working the next step of the hierarchy with the child in the isolated setting. The speech-language pathologist doesn't have to be the contact person, but might be most educated about monitoring communicative pressure to accomplish desensitization. Teachers, psychol-ogists, social workers, and school nurses can serve as the primary trust person to establish a comfort level with the child.

The primary steps in the hierarchy and general principles for intervention are summarized below. Remember that activities must be fun, motivating, and desirable. Desensitization is based in the classic approach-avoidance conflict. The desire to approach a task and earn the reinforcement must be stronger than avoidance for the child with selective mutism.

Establish a Hierarchy to Desensitize to Communicative Pressure

- Establish a nonverbal interaction comfort level. The goal is to get the child to point, nod his head, write or draw, comply with simple direc-tions, and participate in gross-motor activities. Sample activities could include Simon Says, drawing and painting, playing card/board games, sorting and matching tasks, playground games, making snacks, Hide and Seek, etc. Each time the child participates nonverbally and takes a turn, give a reinforcement.

- Establish comfort with whispered interaction. With young children, it helps to introduce transference of focus to something else at this stage. One idea is to introduce a ghost made from a tongue depressor and tissues. The ghost uses a very soft voice, like blowing softly in the wind. Activities are then done with focus on the ghost rather than the child's face. Each time the child takes a turn with a whispered response, give a reinforcement. It may be necessary to begin at rein-forcing a slight movement in the lips, to an open-mouth posture, to an actual whisper. Progress from a posture to a sound, to single words, to word combinations, to short phrases and sentences. Activities might include object identification, Lotto games, drawing cards and naming them, etc.

- Establish comfort with increasingly complex verbal interaction. The analogy of a car works well at this phase. A car has to stay in the garage unless its motor is turned on. The child has to turn on his motor to receive a reinforcement for participating. Start by rolling a car (or ball) back and forth with simple vowel prolongations. Once the child is comfortable, progress to activities requiring single words, to phrases, to sentences, etc. Activities could include card games (e.g., War, Old Maid, Go Fish), drawing an item and trying to guess what it is, memory games with a carrier phrase (e.g., "I'm going on a trip and packing a . . . .").

• Generalize consistent verbal interaction to all settings. Expectations must generalize beyond the therapy room with consistent application of rewards and consequences. Teachers and parents need to know what the current expectation level is at all times. If a family goes to McDonald's® to eat lunch and the child refuses to whisper to the mother or clerk, then the child doesn't get to eat at McDonald's®! The rest of the family enjoys their meal and perhaps rubs in a bit how good it is! (Just kidding!) One first-grade girl had generalized to all settings except gymnastics. We went to gymnastics class and, unless the child talked to the teacher, she was not allowed to participate in the class. It was the child's last holdout, and once she realized she had more power and control over the situation through verbal rather than nonverbal interaction, she complied.

Speech-Language Deficits

• Use word cards for identification at whisper or voicing levels that target a phoneme the child might be having trouble producing. The isolated practice can indirectly incorporate articulation drill.

• Practice manners and other social rules through role play, re-enacting stories, and reading books, helping the child observe other people. This observation and discussion builds the child's knowledge and confidence in pragmatic areas.

Team Approach

• Keep everyone informed about the level of expectation (i.e., nonverbal, whispered, voiced).

• Provide examples of reinforcements and ways to modify expectations to promote success within a comfort level. For example, when a child is working on whispering in the classroom, the teacher might first let the child whisper to her. Then the teacher could verbalize the child's messages to the rest of the class for a few days before asking the child to whisper directly to the whole class.

- Work with the school psychologist to monitor the need for any additional counseling.

- Pair the child with comfortable peers in your therapy session as a transition to full classroom generalization. Bring friends in to play a game or make a snack before expectations are required in the classroom.

General Therapy Guidelines

- Never proceed to the next step in the hierarchy until the child has achieved a level of desensitization (i.e., is not showing signs of communicative sensitivity).

- Once a child has stabilized at a step in the hierarchy in a controlled therapy setting, generalize it throughout the school setting while working on the next step in the therapy setting. For example, if a child has achieved nonverbal responses (e.g., pointing, head nod, etc.), then while you work on establishing a comfort level with whispering, the expectation throughout the school setting is a nonverbal response. Be persistent in increasing demands.

- Give immediate, concrete, positive reinforcements on a daily basis in each activity. Natural consequences of a game or activity will often suffice.

- The therapy program progression should be enjoyable for the child. Don't apply too much pressure. Use fun, nonthreatening activities that are age appropriate and motivating. Minimize any chance of right or wrong responses; the goal is participation.

- Use carryover activities throughout the program, not just toward completion. Establish confidence and comfort in verbal communication in a variety of unstructured settings.

The speech-language pathologist conducting the desensitization program must become comfortable with silence and nonverbal communication. If the therapist immediately fills in verbally, the child won't feel the silence and pressure to communicate. It is important to learn to "read" the child and know when to hold out for a response and when to back off or remove the pressure. The goal is to build tolerance, not magnify anxiety. Also, structure requests and demands so that the child clearly understands the communicative expectation.

Summary Comments . . . .

Selective mutism usually becomes apparent when a child first enrolls in a preschool setting outside of the home. The typical adjustment period passes, but the child continues to withdraw and say nothing while obviously understanding everything and even participating in some nonverbal activities. Parents may be surprised to hear that the child isn't talking and tell you that their child is just being stubborn. The onset age is between three to five years of age, but referral age is six to seven years of age. This discrepancy results from a lack of knowledge regarding the disorder and what to do about it. It also contributes to solidifying a child's resolve to remain mute in situations outside of the home.

Selective mutism is a fascinating, challenging disorder. It is not difficult to identify, but professionals tend to hesitate in taking the responsibility to initiate intervention. Early identification and systematic desensitization can make a dramatic, expedient difference. The speech-language pathologist is a logical professional to assume responsibility for the disorder and coordinate intervention efforts. It requires a strong, consistent program to battle the strong will of the child. The best advice is to be patient! These children hope they can wear you down and will test you to see if you will hold the line. Do so compassionately and sensitively, and the rewards will be tremendous! Very few of the disorders we encounter offer the possibility for such a dramatic and complete resolution as selective mutism. May the force be with you!

References ·

American Psychiatric Association. *Diagnostic and Statistical Manual of Mental Disorders, Fourth Edition.* Washington, D.C.: American Psychiatric Association, 1994.

Baltaxe, C. "Communication Issues in Selective Mutism." Paper presented at the American Speech-Language-Hearing Association Convention. New Orleans, LA, 1994.

Dow, S., Sonies, B., Sceib, D., Moss, S., and Leonard, H. "Practical Guidelines for the Assessment and Treatment of Selective Mutism." *Journal of the American Academy of Child and Adolescent Psychiatry,* Vol. 34 *(7),* pp. 836-846, 1995.

Harris, H. "Elective Mutism: A Tutorial." *Language, Speech and Hearing Services in the Schools*, Vol. 27, pp. 10-15, 1996.

Toland, S. A Survey of Illinois Speech-Language Pathologists and Psychologists Regarding Selective Mutism. Unpublished master's thesis at Eastern Illinois University: Charleston, IL, 1998.

Wright, H., Miller, M., Cook, M., and Littman, J. "Early Identification and Intervention with Children Who Refuse to Speak." *Journal of the American Academy of Child and Adolescent Psychiatry*, Vol. 24, pp. 739-746, 1985.

● ● ● ● ● ● ●

Tourette's Syndrome

Characteristics

- Motor tics
- Vocal tics
- Attention deficit
- Obsessive-compulsive tendencies
- Learning disabilities

- involuntary tics

- short attention span

- high anxiety

- genetic predisposition

- 1/2,000-3,000 males, 1/5,000-10,000 females

- average age at onset 7 years

Syndrome Definition . . . .

Tourette's syndrome has been cited in literature for over a century, but continues to be misunderstood and misdiagnosed to the present day. A French physician named Itard recorded the first medical accounts in 1825, when he described a woman exhibiting severe tics and coprolalia (involuntary swearing). His accounts were reviewed and expanded upon by Gilles de la Tourette, who wrote the first detailed reports on the condition in 1885 and for whom the syndrome is named.

The primary features of Tourette's syndrome are involuntary, multiple motor and vocal tics. A *tic* is defined as "a sudden, rapid, recurrent, nonrhythmic, stereotyped motor movement or vocalization" (*Diagnostic and Statistical Manual of Mental Disorders, Fourth Edition*, 1994). Tics will be further defined in the next section of this chapter. Additional identifying features can include obsessive tendencies, a short attention span, and high anxiety. These characteristic symptoms fluctuate over time, with onset during youth, peak during adolescence, and persistence throughout the lifetime. The bizarre features can be very debilitating socially; emotional problems often develop secondarily to the primary disability. No cure exists; medication and counseling are used to cope with syndrome characteristics.

Incidence figures are higher among males than females, with males afflicted approximately three times more frequently than females. General incidence figures for Tourette's syndrome are one in every 2,500—males range from one in every 2,000-3,000; females range from one in every 5,000-10,000 (Gilbert). The disability is cited in all ethnic groups worldwide. Research suggests that a genetic predisposition for Tourette's syndrome is inherited as an autosomal (non-sex chromosome) dominant condition. A male inheriting the predisposition gene has a 99% chance of developing symptoms; a female has a 70% chance.

The *Diagnostic and Statistical Manual of Mental Disorders, Fourth Edition,* (1994) includes Tourette's Syndrome under Axis I—clinical disorders usually first diagnosed in infancy, childhood, or adolescence: Tic Disorders. The age of onset varies from 2 through 18, with an average onset of age 7. Diagnostic criteria delineated in the *DSM-IV* are summarized in the following chart.

Diagnostic Criteria for Tourette's Syndrome

- Multiple motor tics AND one or more vocal tics are present.

- Tics occur with high daily frequency or intermittently for over one year without the person ever being free of tics for more than three months.

- Symptoms cause significant problems in social, emotional, or occupational functioning.

- The onset is before age 18 years of age.

- Symptoms are not due to other medical conditions or substances.

Behavioral Characteristics Profile . . . .

Tourette's syndrome is characterized by chronic tics of the face and body accompanied by vocal aberrations, such as bursts of profanity, barking, and noises. Fluctuation in the symptom characteristics presents a challenge to accurate diagnosis. During onset and early years of development within the syndrome, intense disruptive periods may be followed by brief periods of total or partial remission. The erratic course of development complicates accurate identification and can lead to secondary emotional and social problems that become the focus. In young children, onset of many of the behaviors is mis-interpreted as other problems, such as allergies to explain vocal grunts and throat clearing. Primary characteristics associated with Tourette's syndrome are explained in the following section.

Motor Tics

Chronic, multiple, motor tics are the cardinal feature associated with Tourette's syndrome. These involuntary movements of the face, limbs, and body can be further classified as simple (sudden, brief, meaningless) or complex (slower, longer, more purposeful). Simple tics usually develop early in the syndrome progression and are comprised primarily of face and head movements, followed by tics developing in the limbs, trunk, and lower body. Complex tics develop as the individual becomes older, and the characteristics wax and wane over time. Examples of simple motor tics include eye blinks, facial grimacing, shrugging the shoulders, and head and arm jerks. Complex motor tics include facial gestures, grooming habits, jumping, stomping, smelling objects, twirling while walking, and imitating movements of others (echokinesis).

Vocal Tics

Vocal tics usually appear following the onset of motor tics, but they are often more noticeable or disruptive than motor tics. As with motor tics, vocal tics can be classified as simple or complex. Examples of simple vocal tics include throat clearing, grunting, sniffing, barking, tongue clicks, and coughing. Complex vocal tics include palilalia (repeating one's own speech patterns), echolalia (repeating a heard sound, word, or phrase) and coprolalia (using profane, obscene, or socially inappropriate words). The involuntary bursts of profanity or obscene language can be quite disconcerting, especially when uttered by a young child.

Attention Deficit

Associated features of Tourette's syndrome include hyperactivity, dis-tractibility, and impulsivity. Manifestation and diagnosis of attention-deficit hyperactivity disorder (ADHD) or attention-deficit disorder (ADD) may precede actual diagnosis of Tourette's syndrome. A teacher or a parent may notice difficulty concentrating or following directions before becoming aware of simple motor tics. While the exact relationship between Tourette's and ADHD is not currently defined, many individuals will require treatment and focus on both entities. The reduced attention span presents significant challenges within the educational setting. ADD/ADHD also compounds medical treatment issues in the area of pharmacological intervention. Stimulants, such as Ritalin, tend to provoke tics and, therefore, must be administered at very low dosages and monitored carefully.

Obsessive-Compulsive Tendencies

Anxiety attacks are not uncommon for individuals with Tourette's syndrome. An obsession to repeat actions or patterns of behavior perseveratively can become very problematic. Obsessions with certain actions, items, or topics can also occur. Without intervention, an individual can become fixated and obsessed with minute details to the point of becoming nonfunctional. Compulsive tendencies are often a means of coping with obsessive anxiety. The need for sameness or control over situations escalates into compulsive, nonfunctional behavior. When a person with Tourette's syndrome becomes highly anxious in a situation, it can lead to abusive or disruptive behaviors. One example might be obsessive-compulsive picking at skin, resulting in large scabs and scars on the body.

Learning Disabilities

Intellectual performance of individuals with Tourette's syndrome is generally within the normal range. Language-learning disabilities often develop as a result of ADD/ADHD components of the disability. Verbal skills are often better than visual-motor, yet memory and concentration problems can compromise educational performance. Research studies suggest approximately 40% of individuals with Tourette's syndrome have learning problems. Special education services and/or placement is often offered to these students when there are significant learning and behavioral problems in the educational setting. Regular education is possible with adjunct supportive professional services.

Speech-Language Issues . . . .

Issues of concern for the speech-language pathologist focus on abusive vocal tics or vocal aberrations produced by the individual with Tourette's syndrome. The other aspect to evaluate is general language development, particularly conceptual language, due to the high incidence of learning disabilities in this population. Speech-language issues to address are summarized in the following section.

Abusive Vocal Tics

Within Tourette's syndrome, simple vocal tics can occur with sufficient frequency and intensity to abuse the laryngeal structure. For example, a six-year-old client diagnosed with Tourette's was enduring a particularly intense period of throat clearing behavior. While not a significant concern under usual circumstances, his throat clearing was charted at over fifty occurrences in a five-minute sample! Teachers noticed that his voice was becoming hoarse, and he was developing a compulsive pattern within that simple vocal tic behavior. The speech-language pathologist's responsibility was to attempt to address that abusive behavioral pattern and modify it.

Socially-Inappropriate or Disruptive Vocal Noises

Coprolalia (involuntary profanity) can be extremely up-setting to both the individual with Tourette's syndrome and those in the immediate vicinity. Loud barking, grunting, and yelling can be disruptive, but can also be misinterpreted as rude, insolent, or aggressive behavior. Attempts to extinguish the involuntary vocal bursts associated with Tourette's syndrome have generally been unsuccessful. However, many speech-language pathologists, other professionals, and parents have been able to replace or modify some of the vocal tic charac-teristics to something less inappropriate or negative socially.

Expressive Language

Vocal tics do not seem to significantly compromise verbal intelligibility; the tics seem to occur at natural pauses or hesitations in a normal speech rhythm. It is important that the person with Tourette's syndrome try to maintain a normal volume, rate, and rhythm in spite of vocal tics that may occur. Remaining calm and composed should minimize any deficits to prosodic features of expressive language. Content may be compromised if vocal tics occur with intense frequency or consistency. The individual may revert to telegraphic or simple-sentence patterns to avoid multiple interruptions before being able to finish a statement or convey a message.

Receptive Language

Intellectual functioning level has a great impact on general language development. Distractibility, impulsivity, and poor attention can significantly effect understanding of verbally-presented information. Language-processing deficits (inability to attach meaning accurately and efficiently to auditorily-presented information) are typical within the profile of individuals with Tourette's syndrome, who also exhibit learning disabilities.

Intervention Issues . . . .

It is unusual to have a definitive diagnosis of Tourette's syndrome during the time a child is three to five years old; often the behavioral characteristics are just emerging. The early intervention setting may be instrumental in obtaining an accurate identification, based on compiling careful behavioral observations over time. If onset is early and diagnosis has occurred at a preschool level, symptoms are likely to be fairly pronounced.

The speech-language pathologist working with elementary school-aged children will be important in collecting observational data to compile a behavioral profile to support Tourette's syndrome. Vocal tics and behaviors may consistently be present, but in a different form. For example, a teacher may notice grunting noises, but by the time you observe, that behavior may have disappeared, only to be replaced with snorting or barking the next week.

Successful intervention will be somewhat dependent on medication effects and the degree of severity of characteristics within the profile. Fluctuation in the intensity of behavioral characteristics can also complicate remedial efforts. Major goal areas to consider for Tourette's syndrome are summarized in the following information.

Vocal Hygiene

- Introduce good vocal production habits and hygiene to prevent abusive vocal patterns from developing or causing laryngeal damage.

- Encourage the child to hydrate frequently to keep the vocal folds moist. A water bottle with reminders for frequent sips is non-disruptive, functional, and an excellent preventive habit to develop.

- Teach vocal relaxation and breathing techniques to prevent tense vocal cords and verbal bursts on residual air.

Vocal Tic Modification

- Introduce replacement vocal behaviors that are less stressful to the organic structures, such as a whistle or noisemaker to replace vocal abusive noises.

- Shape or modify vocal tics to less abusive or disruptive behaviors, such as modifying loud barking to quiet meowing or nasal snorting/grunting to humming.

- Combine good hygiene with reduction of vocal abuse. For example, the little boy mentioned earlier in the chapter who had excessive throat clearing was given a water bottle and told to take a sip of water on every throat-clearing incidence. Eventually he was told to take a sip of water every minute until it had replaced or decreased the throat clearing. Gradually the time was extended between sips without the throat clearing increasing.

Monitor Speech Suprasegmentals

- Evaluate stress in verbal production efforts by informally assessing rate, pitch, rhythm, inflection, and other prosodic features.

- Model and teach a slow, relaxed pattern for producing speech, emphasizing gentle onset of vocalization.

Receptive and Expressive Language Development and Processing

- Evaluate general language comprehension and expression for comparison to developmental age norms.

- Assess language processing, especially the ability to understand abstract language concepts.

- Monitor expressive output to insure that simplification of syntax or content are not occurring to compensate for motor or vocal tics.

- Coordinate with classroom teachers to insure academic success in the classroom through techniques to enhance attention, focus, and minimize impulsive responding.

Team Approach

- A special education teacher can assist in remediating language-based learning disabilities in the educational curriculum and classroom modifications.

- An occupational therapist can monitor fine-motor development for skills such as handwriting, grooming, and any skin hypersensitivities or hyposensitivities.

- A physical therapist can monitor gross-motor development and watch for awkward body postures or clumsiness.

- A psychologist or psychiatrist can provide counseling to cope with secondary personal issues of low self-esteem, social isolation, mis-directed anger, depression, etc.

- A physician can assist in monitoring the efficacy of medication and be alert for potential side effects.

Summary Comments . . . .

Tourette's syndrome can be very difficult to identify and diagnose in young children. Many of the bizarre characteristics are interpreted as willful, manipulative behavior on the part of the individual. A normal IQ contributes to the child's frustration and confusion, often resulting in emotional distress. A child may attempt to cover up motor or vocal tics with immature behavior. Parents are often embarrassed and frustrated by the behavioral profile, which escalates through elementary school, peaking during adolescence.

Dominant characteristics include motor tics of the face, head, and body; vocal tics; obsessive-compulsive tendencies; and attention-deficit hyperactivity disorder. Males are three times more likely to demonstrate the syndrome, with an incidence of approximately one per 2,500. The intensity and frequency of symptoms fluctuate with periodic remissions.

The primary intervention for Tourette's syndrome is pharmacological treatment. Medication can address the motor and vocal tics, obsessive-compulsive tendencies, and attention-deficit components to some extent; however, side effects and drug interactions can be problematic. Haldol (Haloperidol) is the most frequently prescribed medication, but has strong side effects and can become addictive. Stimulant prescriptions to control ADD/ADHD can result in increasing the magnitude of tics. For these reasons, some adults chose to manage the symptom characteristics on their own and opt not to use medication.

Tourette's syndrome is not life-threatening; social, educational, and vocational impact varies based the severity of the symptoms and the ability of the person to cope with the unusual behavioral characteristics.

•   •   •   •   •   •   •

References

American Psychiatric Association. *Diagnostic and Statistical Manual of Mental Disorders, Fourth Edition.* Washington, D.C.: American Psychiatric Association, 1994.

Gilbert, P. *The A-Z Reference Book of Syndromes and Inherited Disorders, Second Edition.* London, England: Chapman & Hall, 1996.

Parker-Fischer, S. and Wasson, M. "A Symposium on Specific Syndromes & Disorders." Workshop presentation at Sarah Bush Lincoln Health Center Education Center: Mattoon, IL, 1996.

Williams Syndrome

Characteristics

- "Elfin" facial features; dental abnormalities
- Physical abnormalities
- Feeding problems
- Excessively social
- Some degree of intellectual disability
- Behaviors related to educational planning
- Motor and perceptual disorders
- Strength in expressive language

- rare, genetic condition

- 1/20,000 live births

- affects males and females equally

- developmental and medical problems

- "cocktail party" speech

Syndrome Definition . . . .

Williams syndrome is a rare, genetic condition that causes medical and developmental problems. At one time it was called *supravalvular aortic stenosis syndrome*, based on the heart defects associated with the condition. It has also been referred to as a *neurobehavioral congenital disorder* that is not due to medical, environmental, or psychosocial factors. This condition occurs in approximately one in 20,000 births, and there are somewhere between 5,000 to 6,000 individuals in the United States with Williams syndrome (Bill, 1998). Williams syndrome can occur in all ethnic groups and is identified in countries throughout the world.

Williams syndrome was first recognized in 1961 as a distinct disorder that is present at birth and affects males and females equally. The cause of Williams syndrome is missing genetic materials on chromosome 7, including the gene that makes the protein elastin, a protein which provides strength and elasticity to vessel walls. The elastin deletion is thought to be present in 95-98% of persons with Williams syndrome.

The clinical diagnosis of Williams syndrome can be confirmed by a blood test in a technique known as *fluorescent in situ hybridization* (FISH). This test of the DNA detects the gene deletion for elastin on chromosome 7, which would be stated "deletion 7q11.23 encompassing elastin gene" (Shprintzen, 1997). This test is readily available at major hospitals throughout the United States.

A late diagnosis or misdiagnosis of Williams syndrome can be a matter of concern, due to the various medical problems that may be associated with Williams syndrome, some of which may be progressive. Each person with Williams syndrome has a unique medical profile. It is likely that the elastin gene deletion accounts for many of the physical features of Williams syndrome.

Behavioral Characteristics Profile

The behavioral characteristics associated with Williams syndrome are explained in the following section.

"Elfin" Facial Features

The characteristic facial features of Williams syndrome have been referred to as "elfin" and become more apparent with age. Facial features include a small upturned nose, a long philtrum (upper lip length), a wide mouth, full lips, and puffiness around the eyes. Persons with Williams syndrome who have blue or green eyes may present a white, lacy "stellate" or "starburst" pattern on their irises (Shprintzen, 1997; Monkaba, 1997). Visual problems may occur, including hyperopia and scoliosis strabismus (Shprintzen, 1997).

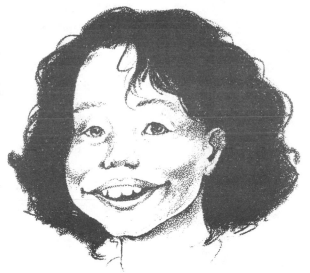

Dental abnormalities, such as slightly small, widely-spaced teeth with small roots and abnormalities of occlusion, are common. Microdontia and enamel hypoplasia are both noted, as well as a shortening of the ramus of the mandible (Shprintzen, 1997).

Physical Abnormalities

Other physical characteristics include kidney abnormalities in structure and function, inguinal and umbilical hernias, and hypercalcemia (elevated blood-calcium levels). The hypercalcemia is thought to cause extreme irritability or the "colicky" symptoms observed in children with Williams syndrome. Heart and blood-vessel problems, such as narrowing of the aorta or pulmonary arteries, are common, as is hypertension. Musculo-skeletal problems, such as low muscle tone and joint looseness, are exhibited, and joint stiffness or contractures can develop. Short stature and microcephaly have also been noted.

Feeding Problems

In infancy, children with Williams syndrome may have low birth weight and may be so slow to gain weight that they are diagnosed as "failure to thrive." Feeding problems are common and may be due to low muscle tone, severe gag reflex, poor suck/swallow, or tactile defensiveness. These feeding problems can resolve as children get older. Irritability (colicky) behavior is exhibited during the middle segment of the infancy period. Delayed development in sitting, crawling, toileting, talking, and walking has been noted.

Excessively Social

In terms of behavior, children with Williams syndrome are excessively social (overly friendly), particularly with adults. They are reported to be outgoing, extremely polite, unafraid of strangers, helpful, cooperative, and eager to please. Adult contact seems to interest children with Williams syndrome more than contact with their peers.

Intellectual Disability

There is some degree of intellectual disability associated with Williams syndrome. Udwin and Yule (1988) report a range of learning difficulties running from mild to severe. They found that 55% of the children were considered severely mentally disabled and 41% were considered moderately mentally disabled. Only 4% of the children in their survey were within the average range of ability. Paul (1995) also notes that Williams syndrome leads to mental retardation, affecting language development.

Speech-Language Issues

- Articulation and Voice

- Language

- Hearing

Behaviors Related to Educational Planning

Overactivity, limited concentration span, and distractibility have all been observed in individuals with Williams syndrome. Monkaba (1997) reports that the distractibility noted in mid-childhood improved with age. Preoccupation with objects or topics, apprehension about change, excessive anxiety and worry, and fearfulness of heights and uneven surfaces are other behaviors noted in persons with Williams syndrome. Some of the fear of heights has been attributed to motor and perceptual disorders (Udwin & Yule, 1988). Although a deficiency in fine motor and spatial relationships has been noted, areas of strength include speech, long-term memory, and social skills. Increased rates of sleep disturbance are also noted (Einfeld et al., 1997), as are difficulties in modulating emotions (Sorrell, 1996).

Speech-Language Issues . . . .

The speech-language pathologist should be aware of several specific aspects of the communication profile in Williams syndrome. These aspects are summarized in the following information.

Articulation and Voice

Speech-language features of Williams syndrome are quite distinct. Relatively good verbal abilities and fluent, articulate speech is apparent by kindergarten. Voice resonance in children with Williams syndrome is usually within normal limits, though some hoarse vocal quality may occur.

Language

Other speech-language characteristics are echolalia, over-talkativeness, and a friendly "cocktail party" manner of conversation. This phenomena is exhibited as incessant chatter at a superficial level with complex, syntactically

Intervention Issues

PRESCHOOL

- Language Stimulation

- Music and Fingerplays

- Family-Centered
  Approach

SCHOOL AGE

- Attention

- Hearing

- Pragmatics

- Word Finding

- Team Approach

correct sentences; long words with sophisticated vocabulary; stereotyped phrases; clichés; and a somewhat perseverative nature. The children exhibiting "cocktail party" manner of speech may seem advanced in expressive language, but may not have the receptive skills to support such an advanced level of language. Word-finding difficulties have also been identified, and the use of circumlocution has been reported (Levine, 1997). There can be a considerable gap between verbal and nonverbal abilities.

Hearing

Hyperacusis (enhanced hearing sensitivity) and aversion to loud noises has been noted in children with Williams syndrome. In addition to this acute sensitivity to sound, many of these children have perfect pitch (Stambaugh, 1996), and they seem to thoroughly enjoy music. Auditory memory also appears to be a strength in children with Williams syndrome.

Intervention Issues . . . .

Preschool

In the preschool years, when developmental milestones in speech language may be delayed, language stimulation is indicated. Possible issues and goals are summarized below.

Language Stimulation

- Increase the child's vocabulary and comprehension of nouns, verbs, descriptors, locatives, etc., based on semantically-related categories.

- A structured setting might be best, due to distractibility and attention difficulties.

- Use behavior management techniques, including prompting and imitation paired with social reinforcement and praise.

Music and Fingerplays

- Developmentally appropriate use of songs and fingerplays are recommended due to reported interest in music.

- Music and fingerplays can also be considered early socio-communicative games and lend themselves well to caregiver-child interaction.

Family-Centered Approach

- Youngest clients will be served in the context of their family.

- A family-centered approach is called for so that the family has input into the goals and outcomes proposed for their child.

- Include the family in service plans to promote generalization of goals into the daily routine.

School Age

When the child begins school, communication difficulties may manifest themselves in a new light. As expressive language strength develops, keep in mind the possible receptive deficits. When evaluating and assessing these children, consider the physical characteristics associated with Williams syndrome. One pertinent characteristic would be hyperacusis, which would call for evaluating in a quiet environment. Also consider visual, cognitive, motor, and attention characteristics in the evaluative process. Looking at the "whole" child will aid in developing a functional communicative program. Use simplified speech to increase the comprehension of language in our patients with Williams syndrome in evaluating as well as in providing intervention.

Keep in mind that the verbal/nonverbal gap in abilities may be the overriding concern in communication therapies with children with Williams syndrome. It is natural to presuppose that these children have excellent language skills due to the high level of expressive language demonstrated, but always check for the receptive component. The underlying foundation concepts may not be in place and may need to be targeted for each child.

The speech-language pathologist working in the school setting should be aware of the possible intervention goals for the child with Williams syndrome. Many of these children will be educated in inclusive settings and may be one of the many students served on an educational caseload. Pragmatic therapy is so important in this population and can be fun for the clinician and the child. Pragmatic intervention also lends itself most favorably to group intervention, which is the format usually seen in a school setting. Targeting socially appropriate use of language in a variety of contexts can incorporate role-play, dramatic creativity, joint action routines, and other functional, enjoyable encounters.

Intervention issues and goals for this population are summarized below.

Attention

- Minimize distractions to help the child attend to pertinent information.

- Use behavior-management techniques such as positive reinforcement for desired behaviors.

- Ignore unwanted behaviors.

- Use stickers and other tangible and token reinforcers, paired with social praise.

Hearing

- Some anxious behaviors associated with Williams syndrome may be associated with hyperacusis (hearing sensitivity).

- Exposure to a variety of sounds in a controlled environment can assist these children in knowing that certain sounds are caused by environmental sources and many of these can be predictable. The phone ringing, school bells, fire alarms, and other sound sources can be identified with the child. Tape record these sounds and play them often for the child to help to break down defensive responses to the sounds.

Pragmatics

- Increase socially-appropriate speech.

- Decrease socially-inappropriate speech. Speech may be utilized more as a means for social contact and to ensure attention than in a communicative role. Ignoring can be a strong therapeutic strategy in this case.

- Redirect the child toward a more appropriate or relevant topic.

- Guide the child to stay on topic for an appropriate number of turns.

- Due to the love of music observed in many children with Williams syndrome, use songs and music in language learning, particularly for pragmatic purposes.

- Children with Williams syndrome may perservate on a topic that particularly interests them. A child with this syndrome can be very adept at guiding any conversation to the topic of his particular interest. Levine (1997) suggests incorporating that favorite interest into the curriculum as a theme or curriculum topic, perhaps in a "whole language" approach. This approach could highly motivate the child. Levine also suggests using role-play, stories, and small groups to expand the child's repertoire of appropriate topics.

- Another pragmatic issue to consider deals with asking and answering questions relevantly. Since many children with Williams syndrome have a perservative style to their language, they may repeat the same questions over and over. Udwin and Yule (1988) suggest insisting that the child repeat an answer that was just given to a question if he asks the same question again. They also suggest that a rule be made that a question is answered one time, and all repetitive questions ignored following that first answer.

Word Finding

- Use cueing systems.

- Phonemic cueing (providing the first phoneme of a targeted word) can key into some of the noted auditory strengths in children with Williams syndrome.

- Visualization can also be used, prompting the child to "picture" the targeted word as a means to accessing the word.

- Semantic cueing, providing a "hint" about the word, might also be attempted.

Team Approach

- A team approach to intervention for children with Williams syndrome is highly recommended.

- An audiologist and an occupational therapist would be primary team members along with the speech-language pathologist to consider communication abilities and perceptual issues.

- The family and the child's teachers would also be valuable members on an intervention team.

Summary Comments . . . .

Williams syndrome is a rare genetic condition with various medical problems exhibited in individuals affected. Children with Williams syndrome have distinctive facial characteristics and often exhibit "cocktail party" speech. Other associated speech-language characteristics include echolalia, over-talkativeness, and hyperacusis. Working with children with Williams syndrome can be a challenge, but they can also prove to be delightful inter-actional partners in speech-language intervention. Working through the strengths exhibited in each individual child to address the needs of that child will evolve into a beneficial therapeutic situation.

References . . . .

Bill, P. "Williams: Rare Syndrome Brings Charm, Challenges." *Pacesetter*, Spring, pp. 5-8, 1998.

Einfeld, S., Tonge, B. J., and Florio, T. "Behavioral and Emotional Disturbance in Individuals with Williams Syndrome." *American Journal on Mental Retardation*, Vol. 102, pp. 45-53, 1997.

Levine, K. "Williams Syndrome: Information for Teachers," July 15, 1998. [Online]. Available: http://www.williams-syndrome.org/

Levine, K. "Guidelines for Psychological Assessment of Young Children (age 4-12) with Williams Syndrome," July 15, 1998. [Online]. Available: http://www.williams-syndrome.org/

Monkaba, T. "Welcome to the Williams Syndrome Association," July 15, 1998. [Online]. Available: http://www.williams-syndrome.org/

Paul, R. *Language Disorders from Infancy to Adolescents: Assessment and Intervention*. St. Louis, MO: Mosby-Year Book Inc., 1995.

Shprintzen, R. J. *Genetics, Syndromes and Communication Disorders*. San Diego, CA: Singular Publishing Group, Inc., 1997.

Sorrell, A. L. "Williams Syndrome: A Family's Journey." Paper presented at the Annual International Conference on Mental Retardation and Developmental Disabilities: Austin, TX, 1996.

Stambaugh, L. "Special Learners with Special Abilities." *Music Educators Journal*, Vol. 83, pp. 19-23, 1996.

Udwin, O., and Yule, W. "Guidelines for Teachers of Children with Williams Syndrome," July 15, 1998. [Online]. Available: http://www.williams-syndrome.org/

Conclusion

" The noblest question in the world is 'What good may I do in it?'"
Benjamin Franklin

This book began with a comment from Benjamin Franklin, so it is only appropriate to allow him to bring us to closure. At the outset, his words challenged us to keep our minds open to new knowledge. The challenge presented by special needs children can be rather overwhelming to professionals. The information explosion sometimes provides too much information, bogging us down in detail. Yet wisdom is fostered through achieving a comfort with knowledge that allows a certain confidence when acting on that knowledge. A composite chart is provided on pages 146-147 to visually summarize the primary points across the 13 disorders addressed in *The Source for Syndromes*.

Words alone do not always make a significant difference. Recitation of facts and knowledge regarding a disability doesn't always translate into effective intervention. The driving force to make a difference in an individual's life is the motivation that lies behind the efforts. This book, hopefully, has addressed some basic questions on the disorders included; your knowledge should have been expanded, yet still be focused. Not all of your questions have been answered, and some of the information probably generated even more questions! But have you attained wisdom?

Webster defines wisdom as "applied learning based on sensible judgment." Therefore, your mission, should you decide to accept it, is to take the knowledge gained from this book and apply it to make sound treatment decisions. Simple words, complex task!

That's where Mr. Franklin helps us out again. We must possess the desire to make a difference in a young person's life. A professional must be motivated to accomplish good things; to improve the quality of life for a child diagnosed with a syndrome disorder. We don't have all the answers; no one does. But sincere efforts to apply learning are a noble gesture by the professional.

The nebulous quality that facilitates a transition from knowledge to wisdom is attitude. Attitude is difficult to define but extremely important in how a professional approaches a child with a disability. A real-life example illustrates this idea quite well.

The mother of a young boy with Asperger's syndrome found the note on the following page in her son's backpack at the end of day. The names have been changed to protect the innocent, but no other editing has occurred!

The Source for Syndromes   142   Copyright © 1999 LinguiSystems, Inc.

10-8-96

Dear Mrs. Parent,

Today at lunch, Alex threw his juice all over a first grader sitting across the table from him because he didn't want to hear her talking to him. Because this is not acceptable behavior, Alex sat "time out" in the front hall with Mrs. James, the teacher on lunch room duty during the incident.

Since Alex didn't get his work finished (from a.m.), at noon recess because of his "time out," I insisted he stay in his second recess to do his assignments. Also, I didn't allow him to attend art when the rest of the class went today. Instead he stayed in the classroom and did some more of his a.m. work.

If he "insists" on "not doing" his assignments (as he has done all day today), I cannot give him grades and this will eventually result in failure of second grade.

Please sign this note and return. Thank you.

> *Sincerely,*
> *Mrs. Teacher*

The boy's mother was quite upset after reading this note. The child was in a normal classroom and had excellent potential to function successfully in that setting. She decided to deal with the note's content to help him understand consequences for his actions.

Her first step was to ask her son who the juice was thrown on. Her son protested that he didn't throw his juice, but she insisted that was not a topic for discussion. Who was the first grader? The boy named a friend who lived in the neighborhood, so the mother told him she was taking her son to apologize. Such a novel idea—an apology for an action rather than time-out! We wonder why the teacher didn't think of that, but we digress! They went to the house and rang the bell. The girl's mother answered and called her daughter to the door. When the little girl appeared and the boy began to apologize, the little girl started crying! When the girl's mother asked what was wrong, the girl responded, "Alex got in so much trouble at school today and it wasn't his fault; he didn't do anything wrong!" Further explanation determined that when Alex began to open his juice box, the girl offered to help because she knew Alex had fine-motor problems (from the Asperger's syndrome). He responded that "No, I want to do it myself." That comment is the one that the teacher interpreted as "he didn't want to hear her talking."

Well, the fine-motor deficits and desire to independently open and insert the straw resulted in too much pressure, and—you guessed it—juice squirted out. The teacher's interpretation was "he threw his juice all over her." His mom was relieved that the incident had been accidental, but worried that the teacher hadn't explored what had really happened. But the lunchroom is busy; maybe she could talk with the teacher tomorrow.

Mrs. Parent knew that Alex would only drink red juice and offered to launder or replace the girl's clothes. The girl's mother said she was wearing the clothes she had worn to school. The girl volunteered that the juice didn't get on her clothes, but on the linoleum floor! Again, a different interpretation. Rather than clean up the accident, the teacher's solution was to put the boy in time-out and take away recess, consequences far removed from natural learning.

The second paragraph of the teacher's note is alarming. The morning work apparently caused an anxiety response in the boy that was refreshed all day by continually introducing it. Activities that could reduce anxiety (recess and art) were removed, and the anxiety stimulus was presented as a replacement. This teacher was making sure that the child in her classroom with a disability had a terrible day and was continually singled out for behavioral problems. In fact, the teacher was creating many of the behavior problems!

The last paragraph inadvertently reveals the teacher's attitude. In Mrs. Teacher's mind, this child has already failed second grade, even though it is only the first week of October. She is not comfortable with either the disability or the child and is insuring his failure in the regular classroom setting. Mrs. Parent shared with the speech-language pathologist that the teacher had suggested she visit the behavior-disordered classroom as a possible placement for Alex. While not a totally unreasonable suggestion, it occurred during the first week of school, before Alex or any other child-ren had settled into the new setting.

The administrator refused all attempts to in-service, assist, change teachers, etc. Alex had a miserable year and gained very little. By May, he was liter-ally sick from the anxiety of having to attend school and sit in the hallway in "time-out" most of the day, so his mother pulled him out for summer vacation early. Despite protests from the teacher, he was passed to third grade, where a new teacher made all the difference. She fostered his development, tolerated his differences, and challenged his intellect. He set the class standard of achievement in some subjects, never was in time-out, and had a wonderfully productive year. The only change was a teacher—with an attitude!

As a professional, you have these responsibilities in meeting the needs of your students:

1. Learn what you can about the disability.

2. Access in-service training or resources to help you understand the disability and how to intervene effectively. Don't waste time re-inventing the wheel; talk to other professionals and benefit from their experience.

3. See a child, not a syndrome label or medical jargon.

4. Work conscientiously to channel your knowledge into wisdom, using careful, conscientiously applied goals for making a difference in the quality of life.

5. Don't get overwhelmed by the big picture of the future. Begin with the primary areas in which you can make a difference.

Preschool intervention is an exciting time to work with children. The neuro-plasticity of the human body continues to amaze us when remedial efforts are intense, focused, and pertinent. Strive to do your best with a positive attitude, good intentions, and knowledge transformed into confident wisdom.

● ● ● ● ● ● ●

Syndrome Overview

	Angelman	Asperger's	Autism	Down	Fetal Alcohol	Fetal Rubella	Fragile X
Age of Onset	birth	24-36 months	36 months	birth	birth	birth	birth
Cause	genetic (chrom. 15)	neurological	neurological	genetic (chrom. 21)	CNS damage	German measles	genetic (X chrom.)
Incidence	1/10-25,000	1/1-7,000	15/10,000	1/7-800	1/1-2,500		1/1,000 M 1/2,000 F
Deficits/Impairments							
Cognitive	X		X	X	X	X	X
Oral Motor	X		X	X			X
Language Learning	X	X	X	X	X	X	X
Gross/Fine Motor	X	X	X		X		X
Physical/Facial	X			X	X		X
Seizures	X		X				
Social	X	X	X				
Hearing				X	X	X	X
Other Health Issues				X	X	X	
Speech-Language Issues							
Auditory				X	X	X	
Feeding/Swallowing	X				X		X
Language	X	X	X	X	X	X	X
Pragmatics	X	X	X	X			X
Voice/Articulation				X	X		X
Intervention							
Augmentative Commun.	X		X			X	X
Oral Motor/Articulation	X		X	X			X
Social/Pragmatics	X	X	X	X			X
Developmental Language	X		X	X	X	X	X
Abstract Language		X			X		
Aural Rehabilitation				X	X	X	

	Landau-Kleffner	Prader-Willi	Rett's	Selective Mutism	Tourette's	Williams
Age of Onset	3-7 years	birth	2-6 months	3-5 years.	7 years	birth
Cause	neurological	genetic (chrom. 15)	genetic	behavioral	genetic	genetic (chrom. 7)
Incidence	< 500 worldwide	1/8-25,000	1/10-15,000 (F only)	1/1,000	1/2-3,000 M 1/5-10,000 F	1/20,000
Deficits/Impairments						
Cognitive		X	X			X
Oral Motor		X	X			X
Language Learning	X	X	X	X	X	X
Gross/Fine Motor		X	X		X (tics)	X
Physical/Facial		X				X
Seizures	X		X			
Social				X		
Hearing						X
Other Health Issues		X				X
Speech-Language Issues						
Auditory						
Feeding/Swallowing		X	X			X
Language	X	X	X			X
Pragmatics				X	X	
Voice/Articulation	X	X	X		X	X
Intervention						
Augmentative Commun.	X		X			
Oral Motor/Articulation		X	X	X		X
Social/Pragmatics				X	X	X
Developmental Language		X	X			X
Abstract Language	X			X	X	
Aural Rehabilitation						

The Source for Syndromes